Inpatient Obstetric Nurse Exam

SECRETS

Study Guide
Your Key to Exam Success

Inpatient Obstetric Test Review for the
Inpatient Obstetric Nurse Exam

Dear Future Exam Success Story:

First of all, **THANK YOU** for purchasing Mometrix study materials!

Second, congratulations! You are one of the few determined test-takers who are committed to doing whatever it takes to excel on your exam. **You have come to the right place.** We developed these study materials with one goal in mind: to deliver you the information you need in a format that's concise and easy to use.

In addition to optimizing your guide for the content of the test, we've outlined our recommended steps for breaking down the preparation process into small, attainable goals so you can make sure you stay on track.

We've also analyzed the entire test-taking process, identifying the most common pitfalls and showing how you can overcome them and be ready for any curveball the test throws you.

Standardized testing is one of the biggest obstacles on your road to success, which only increases the importance of doing well in the high-pressure, high-stakes environment of test day. Your results on this test could have a significant impact on your future, and this guide provides the information and practical advice to help you achieve your full potential on test day.

Your success is our success

We would love to hear from you! If you would like to share the story of your exam success or if you have any questions or comments in regard to our products, please contact us at **800-673-8175** or **support@mometrix.com**.

Thanks again for your business and we wish you continued success!

Sincerely,
The Mometrix Test Preparation Team

Need more help? Check out our flashcards at:
http://MometrixFlashcards.com/InpatientObstetric

TABLE OF CONTENTS

Introduction

Thank you for purchasing this resource! You have made the choice to prepare yourself for a test that could have a huge impact on your future, and this guide is designed to help you be fully ready for test day. Obviously, it's important to have a solid understanding of the test material, but you also need to be prepared for the unique environment and stressors of the test, so that you can perform to the best of your abilities.

For this purpose, the first section that appears in this guide is the **Secret Keys**. We've devoted countless hours to meticulously researching what works and what doesn't, and we've boiled down our findings to the five most impactful steps you can take to improve your performance on the test. We start at the beginning with study planning and move through the preparation process, all the way to the testing strategies that will help you get the most out of what you know when you're finally sitting in front of the test.

We recommend that you start preparing for your test as far in advance as possible. However, if you've bought this guide as a last-minute study resource and only have a few days before your test, we recommend that you skip over the first two Secret Keys since they address a long-term study plan.

If you struggle with **test anxiety**, we strongly encourage you to check out our recommendations for how you can overcome it. Test anxiety is a formidable foe, but it can be beaten, and we want to make sure you have the tools you need to defeat it.

- 1 -

Secret Key #1 – Plan Big, Study Small

There's a lot riding on your performance. If you want to ace this test, you're going to need to keep your skills sharp and the material fresh in your mind. You need a plan that lets you review everything you need to know while still fitting in your schedule. We'll break this strategy down into three categories.

Information Organization

Start with the information you already have: the official test outline. From this, you can make a complete list of all the concepts you need to cover before the test. Organize these concepts into groups that can be studied together, and create a list of any related vocabulary you need to learn so you can brush up on any difficult terms. You'll want to keep this vocabulary list handy once you actually start studying since you may need to add to it along the way.

Time Management

Once you have your set of study concepts, decide how to spread them out over the time you have left before the test. Break your study plan into small, clear goals so you have a manageable task for each day and know exactly what you're doing. Then just focus on one small step at a time. When you manage your time this way, you don't need to spend hours at a time studying. Studying a small block of content for a short period each day helps you retain information better and avoid stressing over how much you have left to do. You can relax knowing that you have a plan to cover everything in time. In order for this strategy to be effective though, you have to start studying early and stick to your schedule. Avoid the exhaustion and futility that comes from last-minute cramming!

Study Environment

The environment you study in has a big impact on your learning. Studying in a coffee shop, while probably more enjoyable, is not likely to be as fruitful as studying in a quiet room. It's important to keep distractions to a minimum. You're only planning to study for a short block of time, so make the most of it. Don't pause to check your phone or get up to find a snack. It's also important to **avoid multitasking**. Research has consistently shown that multitasking will make your studying dramatically less effective. Your study area should also be comfortable and well-lit so you don't have the distraction of straining your eyes or sitting on an uncomfortable chair.

The time of day you study is also important. You want to be rested and alert. Don't wait until just before bedtime. Study when you'll be most likely to comprehend and remember. Even better, if you know what time of day your test will be, set that time aside for study. That way your brain will be used to working on that subject at that specific time and you'll have a better chance of recalling information.

Finally, it can be helpful to team up with others who are studying for the same test. Your actual studying should be done in as isolated an environment as possible, but the work of organizing the information and setting up the study plan can be divided up. In between study sessions, you can discuss with your teammates the concepts that you're all studying and quiz each other on the details. Just be sure that your teammates are as serious about the test as you are. If you find that your study time is being replaced with social time, you might need to find a new team.

Secret Key #2 – Make Your Studying Count

You're devoting a lot of time and effort to preparing for this test, so you want to be absolutely certain it will pay off. This means doing more than just reading the content and hoping you can remember it on test day. It's important to make every minute of study count. There are two main areas you can focus on to make your studying count:

Retention

It doesn't matter how much time you study if you can't remember the material. You need to make sure you are retaining the concepts. To check your retention of the information you're learning, try recalling it at later times with minimal prompting. Try carrying around flashcards and glance at one or two from time to time or ask a friend who's also studying for the test to quiz you.

To enhance your retention, look for ways to put the information into practice so that you can apply it rather than simply recalling it. If you're using the information in practical ways, it will be much easier to remember. Similarly, it helps to solidify a concept in your mind if you're not only reading it to yourself but also explaining it to someone else. Ask a friend to let you teach them about a concept you're a little shaky on (or speak aloud to an imaginary audience if necessary). As you try to summarize, define, give examples, and answer your friend's questions, you'll understand the concepts better and they will stay with you longer. Finally, step back for a big picture view and ask yourself how each piece of information fits with the whole subject. When you link the different concepts together and see them working together as a whole, it's easier to remember the individual components.

Finally, practice showing your work on any multi-step problems, even if you're just studying. Writing out each step you take to solve a problem will help solidify the process in your mind, and you'll be more likely to remember it during the test.

Modality

Modality simply refers to the means or method by which you study. Choosing a study modality that fits your own individual learning style is crucial. No two people learn best in exactly the same way, so it's important to know your strengths and use them to your advantage.

For example, if you learn best by visualization, focus on visualizing a concept in your mind and draw an image or a diagram. Try color-coding your notes, illustrating them, or creating symbols that will trigger your mind to recall a learned concept. If you learn best by hearing or discussing information, find a study partner who learns the same way or read aloud to yourself. Think about how to put the information in your own words. Imagine that you are giving a lecture on the topic and record yourself so you can listen to it later.

For any learning style, flashcards can be helpful. Organize the information so you can take advantage of spare moments to review. Underline key words or phrases. Use different colors for different categories. Mnemonic devices (such as creating a short list in which every item starts with the same letter) can also help with retention. Find what works best for you and use it to store the information in your mind most effectively and easily.

Secret Key #3 – Practice the Right Way

Your success on test day depends not only on how many hours you put into preparing, but also on whether you prepared the right way. It's good to check along the way to see if your studying is paying off. One of the most effective ways to do this is by taking practice tests to evaluate your progress. Practice tests are useful because they show exactly where you need to improve. Every time you take a practice test, pay special attention to these three groups of questions:

- The questions you got wrong
- The questions you had to guess on, even if you guessed right
- The questions you found difficult or slow to work through

This will show you exactly what your weak areas are, and where you need to devote more study time. Ask yourself why each of these questions gave you trouble. Was it because you didn't understand the material? Was it because you didn't remember the vocabulary? Do you need more repetitions on this type of question to build speed and confidence? Dig into those questions and figure out how you can strengthen your weak areas as you go back to review the material.

Additionally, many practice tests have a section explaining the answer choices. It can be tempting to read the explanation and think that you now have a good understanding of the concept. However, an explanation likely only covers part of the question's broader context. Even if the explanation makes sense, **go back and investigate** every concept related to the question until you're positive you have a thorough understanding.

As you go along, keep in mind that the practice test is just that: practice. Memorizing these questions and answers will not be very helpful on the actual test because it is unlikely to have any of the same exact questions. If you only know the right answers to the sample questions, you won't be prepared for the real thing. **Study the concepts** until you understand them fully, and then you'll be able to answer any question that shows up on the test.

It's important to wait on the practice tests until you're ready. If you take a test on your first day of study, you may be overwhelmed by the amount of material covered and how much you need to learn. Work up to it gradually.

On test day, you'll need to be prepared for answering questions, managing your time, and using the test-taking strategies you've learned. It's a lot to balance, like a mental marathon that will have a big impact on your future. Like training for a marathon, you'll need to start slowly and work your way up. When test day arrives, you'll be ready.

Start with the strategies you've read in the first two Secret Keys—plan your course and study in the way that works best for you. If you have time, consider using multiple study resources to get different approaches to the same concepts. It can be helpful to see difficult concepts from more than one angle. Then find a good source for practice tests. Many times, the test website will suggest potential study resources or provide sample tests.

Practice Test Strategy

When you're ready to start taking practice tests, follow this strategy:

1. Take the first test with no time constraints and with your notes and study guide handy. Take your time and focus on applying the strategies you've learned.
2. Take the second practice test open-book as well, but set a timer and practice pacing yourself to finish in time.
3. Take any other practice tests as if it were test day. Set a timer and put away your study materials. Sit at a table or desk in a quiet room, imagine yourself at the testing center, and answer questions as quickly and accurately as possible.
4. Keep repeating step 3 on a regular basis until you run out of practice tests or it's time for the actual test. Your mind will be ready for the schedule and stress of test day, and you'll be able to focus on recalling the material you've learned.

Secret Key #4 – Pace Yourself

Once you're fully prepared for the material on the test, your biggest challenge on test day will be managing your time. Just knowing that the clock is ticking can make you panic even if you have plenty of time left. Work on pacing yourself so you can build confidence against the time constraints of the exam. Pacing is a difficult skill to master, especially in a high-pressure environment, so **practice is vital**.

Set time expectations for your pace based on how much time is available. For example, if a section has 60 questions and the time limit is 30 minutes, you know you have to average 30 seconds or less per question in order to answer them all. Although 30 seconds is the hard limit, set 25 seconds per question as your goal, so you reserve extra time to spend on harder questions. When you budget extra time for the harder questions, you no longer have any reason to stress when those questions take longer to answer.

Don't let this time expectation distract you from working through the test at a calm, steady pace, but keep it in mind so you don't spend too much time on any one question. Recognize that taking extra time on one question you don't understand may keep you from answering two that you do understand later in the test. If your time limit for a question is up and you're still not sure of the answer, mark it and move on, and come back to it later if the time and the test format allow. If the testing format doesn't allow you to return to earlier questions, just make an educated guess; then put it out of your mind and move on.

On the easier questions, be careful not to rush. It may seem wise to hurry through them so you have more time for the challenging ones, but it's not worth missing one if you know the concept and just didn't take the time to read the question fully. Work efficiently but make sure you understand the question and have looked at all of the answer choices, since more than one may seem right at first.

Even if you're paying attention to the time, you may find yourself a little behind at some point. You should speed up to get back on track, but do so wisely. Don't panic; just take a few seconds less on each question until you're caught up. Don't guess without thinking, but do look through the answer choices and eliminate any you know are wrong. If you can get down to two choices, it is often worthwhile to guess from those. Once you've chosen an answer, move on and don't dwell on any that you skipped or had to hurry through. If a question was taking too long, chances are it was one of the harder ones, so you weren't as likely to get it right anyway.

On the other hand, if you find yourself getting ahead of schedule, it may be beneficial to slow down a little. The more quickly you work, the more likely you are to make a careless mistake that will affect your score. You've budgeted time for each question, so don't be afraid to spend that time. Practice an efficient but careful pace to get the most out of the time you have.

Secret Key #5 – Have a Plan for Guessing

When you're taking the test, you may find yourself stuck on a question. Some of the answer choices seem better than others, but you don't see the one answer choice that is obviously correct. What do you do?

The scenario described above is very common, yet most test takers have not effectively prepared for it. Developing and practicing a plan for guessing may be one of the single most effective uses of your time as you get ready for the exam.

In developing your plan for guessing, there are three questions to address:

- When should you start the guessing process?
- How should you narrow down the choices?
- Which answer should you choose?

When to Start the Guessing Process

Unless your plan for guessing is to select C every time (which, despite its merits, is not what we recommend), you need to leave yourself enough time to apply your answer elimination strategies. Since you have a limited amount of time for each question, that means that if you're going to give yourself the best shot at guessing correctly, you have to decide quickly whether or not you will guess.

Of course, the best-case scenario is that you don't have to guess at all, so first, see if you can answer the question based on your knowledge of the subject and basic reasoning skills. Focus on the key words in the question and try to jog your memory of related topics. Give yourself a chance to bring the knowledge to mind, but once you realize that you don't have (or you can't access) the knowledge you need to answer the question, it's time to start the guessing process.

It's almost always better to start the guessing process too early than too late. It only takes a few seconds to remember something and answer the question from knowledge. Carefully eliminating wrong answer choices takes longer. Plus, going through the process of eliminating answer choices can actually help jog your memory.

Summary: Start the guessing process as soon as you decide that you can't answer the question based on your knowledge.

How to Narrow Down the Choices

The next chapter in this book (**Test-Taking Strategies**) includes a wide range of strategies for how to approach questions and how to look for answer choices to eliminate. You will definitely want to read those carefully, practice them, and figure out which ones work best for you. Here though, we're going to address a mindset rather than a particular strategy.

Your chances of guessing an answer correctly depend on how many options you are choosing from.

How many choices you have	How likely you are to guess correctly
5	20%
4	25%
3	33%
2	50%
1	100%

You can see from this chart just how valuable it is to be able to eliminate incorrect answers and make an educated guess, but there are two things that many test takers do that cause them to miss out on the benefits of guessing:

- Accidentally eliminating the correct answer
- Selecting an answer based on an impression

We'll look at the first one here, and the second one in the next section.

To avoid accidentally eliminating the correct answer, we recommend a thought exercise called **the $5 challenge**. In this challenge, you only eliminate an answer choice from contention if you are willing to bet $5 on it being wrong. Why $5? Five dollars is a small but not insignificant amount of money. It's an amount you could afford to lose but wouldn't want to throw away. And while losing $5 once might not hurt too much, doing it twenty times will set you back $100. In the same way, each small decision you make—eliminating a choice here, guessing on a question there—won't by itself impact your score very much, but when you put them all together, they can make a big difference. By holding each answer choice elimination decision to a higher standard, you can reduce the risk of accidentally eliminating the correct answer.

The $5 challenge can also be applied in a positive sense: If you are willing to bet $5 that an answer choice *is* correct, go ahead and mark it as correct.

Summary: Only eliminate an answer choice if you are willing to bet $5 that it is wrong.

Which Answer to Choose

You're taking the test. You've run into a hard question and decided you'll have to guess. You've eliminated all the answer choices you're willing to bet $5 on. Now you have to pick an answer. Why do we even need to talk about this? Why can't you just pick whichever one you feel like when the time comes?

The answer to these questions is that if you don't come into the test with a plan, you'll rely on your impression to select an answer choice, and if you do that, you risk falling into a trap. The test writers know that everyone who takes their test will be guessing on some of the questions, so they intentionally write wrong answer choices to seem plausible. You still have to pick an answer though, and if the wrong answer choices are designed to look right, how can you ever be sure that you're not falling for their trap? The best solution we've found to this dilemma is to take the decision out of your hands entirely. Here is the process we recommend:

Once you've eliminated any choices that you are confident (willing to bet $5) are wrong, select the first remaining choice as your answer.

Whether you choose to select the first remaining choice, the second, or the last, the important thing is that you use some preselected standard. Using this approach guarantees that you will not be enticed into selecting an answer choice that looks right, because you are not basing your decision on how the answer choices look.

This is not meant to make you question your knowledge. Instead, it is to help you recognize the difference between your knowledge and your impressions. There's a huge difference between thinking an answer is right because of what you know, and thinking an answer is right because it looks or sounds like it should be right.

Summary: To ensure that your selection is appropriately random, make a predetermined selection from among all answer choices you have not eliminated.

Test-Taking Strategies

This section contains a list of test-taking strategies that you may find helpful as you work through the test. By taking what you know and applying logical thought, you can maximize your chances of answering any question correctly!

It is very important to realize that every question is different and every person is different: no single strategy will work on every question, and no single strategy will work for every person. That's why we've included all of them here, so you can try them out and determine which ones work best for different types of questions and which ones work best for you.

Question Strategies

Read Carefully

Read the question and answer choices carefully. Don't miss the question because you misread the terms. You have plenty of time to read each question thoroughly and make sure you understand what is being asked. Yet a happy medium must be attained, so don't waste too much time. You must read carefully, but efficiently.

Contextual Clues

Look for contextual clues. If the question includes a word you are not familiar with, look at the immediate context for some indication of what the word might mean. Contextual clues can often give you all the information you need to decipher the meaning of an unfamiliar word. Even if you can't determine the meaning, you may be able to narrow down the possibilities enough to make a solid guess at the answer to the question.

Prefixes

If you're having trouble with a word in the question or answer choices, try dissecting it. Take advantage of every clue that the word might include. Prefixes and suffixes can be a huge help. Usually they allow you to determine a basic meaning. Pre- means before, post- means after, pro - is positive, de- is negative. From prefixes and suffixes, you can get an idea of the general meaning of the word and try to put it into context.

Hedge Words

Watch out for critical hedge words, such as *likely, may, can, sometimes, often, almost, mostly, usually, generally, rarely*, and *sometimes*. Question writers insert these hedge phrases to cover every possibility. Often an answer choice will be wrong simply because it leaves no room for exception. Be on guard for answer choices that have definitive words such as *exactly* and *always*.

Switchback Words

Stay alert for *switchbacks*. These are the words and phrases frequently used to alert you to shifts in thought. The most common switchback words are *but, although*, and *however*. Others include *nevertheless, on the other hand, even though, while, in spite of, despite, regardless of*. Switchback words are important to catch because they can change the direction of the question or an answer choice.

- 10 -

Face Value

When in doubt, use common sense. Accept the situation in the problem at face value. Don't read too much into it. These problems will not require you to make wild assumptions. If you have to go beyond creativity and warp time or space in order to have an answer choice fit the question, then you should move on and consider the other answer choices. These are normal problems rooted in reality. The applicable relationship or explanation may not be readily apparent, but it is there for you to figure out. Use your common sense to interpret anything that isn't clear.

Answer Choice Strategies

Answer Selection

The most thorough way to pick an answer choice is to identify and eliminate wrong answers until only one is left, then confirm it is the correct answer. Sometimes an answer choice may immediately seem right, but be careful. The test writers will usually put more than one reasonable answer choice on each question, so take a second to read all of them and make sure that the other choices are not equally obvious. As long as you have time left, it is better to read every answer choice than to pick the first one that looks right without checking the others.

Eliminate Answers

Eliminate answer choices as soon as you realize they are wrong, but make sure you consider all possibilities. If you are eliminating answer choices and realize that the last one you are left with is also wrong, don't panic. Start over and consider each choice again. There may be something you missed the first time that you will realize on the second pass.

Avoid Fact Traps

Don't be distracted by an answer choice that is factually true but doesn't answer the question. You are looking for the choice that answers the question. Stay focused on what the question is asking for so you don't accidentally pick an answer that is true but incorrect. Always go back to the question and make sure the answer choice you've selected actually answers the question and is not merely a true statement.

Extreme Statements

In general, you should avoid answers that put forth extreme actions as standard practice or proclaim controversial ideas as established fact. An answer choice that states the "process should be used in certain situations, if..." is much more likely to be correct than one that states the "process should be discontinued completely." The first is a calm rational statement and doesn't even make a definitive, uncompromising stance, using a hedge word *if* to provide wiggle room, whereas the second choice is a radical idea and far more extreme.

Benchmark

As you read through the answer choices and you come across one that seems to answer the question well, mentally select that answer choice. This is not your final answer, but it's the one that will help you evaluate the other answer choices. The one that you selected is your benchmark or standard for judging each of the other answer choices. Every other answer choice must be compared to your benchmark. That choice is correct until proven otherwise by another answer choice beating it. If you find a better answer, then that one becomes your new benchmark. Once

- 11 -

you've decided that no other choice answers the question as well as your benchmark, you have your final answer.

Predict the Answer

Before you even start looking at the answer choices, it is often best to try to predict the answer. When you come up with the answer on your own, it is easier to avoid distractions and traps because you will know exactly what to look for. The right answer choice is unlikely to be word-for-word what you came up with, but it should be a close match. Even if you are confident that you have the right answer, you should still take the time to read each option before moving on.

General Strategies

Tough Questions

If you are stumped on a problem or it appears too hard or too difficult, don't waste time. Move on! Remember though, if you can quickly check for obviously incorrect answer choices, your chances of guessing correctly are greatly improved. Before you completely give up, at least try to knock out a couple of possible answers. Eliminate what you can and then guess at the remaining answer choices before moving on.

Check Your Work

Since you will probably not know every term listed and the answer to every question, it is important that you get credit for the ones that you do know. Don't miss any questions through careless mistakes. If at all possible, try to take a second to look back over your answer selection and make sure you've selected the correct answer choice and haven't made a costly careless mistake (such as marking an answer choice that you didn't mean to mark). This quick double check should more than pay for itself in caught mistakes for the time it costs.

Pace Yourself

It's easy to be overwhelmed when you're looking at a page full of questions; your mind is confused and full of random thoughts, and the clock is ticking down faster than you would like. Calm down and maintain the pace that you have set for yourself. Especially as you get down to the last few minutes of the test, don't let the small numbers on the clock make you panic. As long as you are on track by monitoring your pace, you are guaranteed to have time for each question.

Don't Rush

It is very easy to make errors when you are in a hurry. Maintaining a fast pace in answering questions is pointless if it makes you miss questions that you would have gotten right otherwise. Test writers like to include distracting information and wrong answers that seem right. Taking a little extra time to avoid careless mistakes can make all the difference in your test score. Find a pace that allows you to be confident in the answers that you select.

Keep Moving

Panicking will not help you pass the test, so do your best to stay calm and keep moving. Taking deep breaths and going through the answer elimination steps you practiced can help to break through a stress barrier and keep your pace.

- 12 -

Final Notes

The combination of a solid foundation of content knowledge and the confidence that comes from practicing your plan for applying that knowledge is the key to maximizing your performance on test day. As your foundation of content knowledge is built up and strengthened, you'll find that the strategies included in this chapter become more and more effective in helping you quickly sift through the distractions and traps of the test to isolate the correct answer.

Now it's time to move on to the test content chapters of this book, but be sure to keep your goal in mind. As you read, think about how you will be able to apply this information on the test. If you've already seen sample questions for the test and you have an idea of the question format and style, try to come up with questions of your own that you can answer based on what you're reading. This will give you valuable practice applying your knowledge in the same ways you can expect to on test day.

Good luck and good studying!

Factors Affecting the Fetus and Newborn

Disease Processes Affecting the Fetus and Newborn

Preeclampsia, Eclampsia, and HELLP Syndrome

Preeclampsia is present when a pregnant patient's systolic pressure is greater than 140 mm Hg, the diastolic pressure is greater than 90 mm Hg, and proteinuria is greater than 300 mg per 24 hours or greater than 1 g/L on a dipstick. The woman is considered **preeclamptic** in absence of proteinuria if she has headaches, visual disturbances, pain in the right epigastric or abdominal area, and other lab tests are abnormal. **Eclampsia** occurs when a pregnant women suffers a seizure. Preeclampsia may or may not have been diagnosed previously. There is no other reason for the seizure. **HELLP syndrome**, a serious complication often preceded by preeclampsia, is accompanied by Hemolysis, Elevated Liver enzymes, and Low Platelets. All three of these disorders put the mother and fetus at risk for death.

Risk Factors for Preeclampsia

Mothers younger than 19 years of age and mothers older than 35 years of age are at higher risk. A family history of hypertension caused by pregnancy is a risk factor. African-American women are at higher risk for hypertension in general, and therefore for preeclampsia. Poor diet and tobacco use increase the risk. First pregnancies and the first pregnancy with a new father have higher incidences of preeclampsia. The presence of diabetes or gestational diabetes, metabolic syndrome, renal disease, migraine headaches, or collagen vascular disease increases the risk for preeclampsia, as does a hydatiform mole or fetal hydrops.

Effects of Preeclampsia on Fetus

When preeclampsia is present, the uterus and placenta are invaded by abnormal spiral arteries with a limited ability to dilate. Blood vessels of the uterus and placenta may become necrotic. The entire uteroplacental unit suffers decreased perfusion, which causes fetal compromise. Decreased placental functioning leaves the fetus with few or no reserves for the labor and delivery process. Premature birth may occur. Intrauterine growth retardation, oligohydramnios, abruptio placentae, and intrauterine death can occur. The fetus must be monitored frequently when preeclampsia is present, since compromise can require an early delivery.

Chronic Hypertension and Gestational Hypertension

Chronic hypertension in pregnancy is hypertension that is present before pregnancy occurs, hypertension that occurs before the twentieth week of gestation, or hypertension that persists after 3 months postpartum. The blood pressure is greater than 140/90 mm Hg systolic, diastolic, or both. It puts the pregnancy at risk for placental abruption. Rates of hypertension in pregnancy are increasing overall in women with those of American Indian, Caucasian, and African-American descent at greatest risk. **Gestational hypertension** begins after the twentieth week of gestation. Blood pressure returns to normal before 3 months postpartum. The fetus is affected by decreased blood perfusion and decreased oxygen and nutrients, and may be small for gestational age when born. Preeclampsia does not develop.

Impact of Sexually Transmitted Diseases on Fetus and Newborn

HIV Infection

Most infants infected with **AIDS/HIV** acquire the infection from their mothers (vertical transmission). The perinatal transmission rate is 30% in untreated HIV positive mothers, usually acquired during delivery. Neonates are usually asymptomatic but are at risk for prematurity, low birth weight, and small for gestational age (SGA). Infants may show failure to thrive, hepatomegaly, interstitial lymphocytic pneumonia, recurrent infections, and CNS abnormalities. Optimal treatment reduces the perinatal transmission rate to as low as 1-2%:

- **Antiviral therapy** during the pregnancy: A reduced viral load in the mother lessens the likelihood of prenatal transmission.
- **Elective Caesarian** before the amniotic membranes rupture. **Emergency Caesarian**, rupture of membranes longer than 4 hours, and the need for an episiotomy all increase the likelihood of infection during delivery.
- **Antiviral medications** for the neonate for the first 6 weeks of life. The first dose should be given within the first 6-12 hours after delivery.
- **Avoiding breastfeeding**: The risk of HIV transmission with breastfeeding is 0.7% per month of breastfeeding.

Chlamydia and Human Papillomavirus

While the woman is often asymptomatic, **chlamydia** can affect the pregnancy, increasing the risk of preterm labor, premature rupture of the membranes, and chorioamnionitis. The infant may be infected during delivery, resulting in neonatal conjunctivitis and/or pneumonitis. Erythromycin ophthalmic ointment should be administered as a prophylaxis. **Human papillomavirus** (condylomata acuminata/genital warts) may exacerbate with pregnancy, causing proliferation of lesions, but the usual treatments are contraindicated although lesions may be excised, cauterized, or treated with cryotherapy. The virus can be transmitted to the infant during delivery, resulting in recurrent epithelial tumors in the neonate's mucous membranes and larynx (recurrent respiratory papillomatosis). Caesarean delivery reduces but does not eliminate risk. Neonates may exhibit weak cry, dysphagia, cough, or inspiratory stridor. Children may require multiple surgical interventions until puberty at which time they may experience remission. Routine immunization of preadolescent children is recommended to reduce incidence.

Gonorrhea and Syphilis

Gonorrhea (often associated with chlamydia infection) may cause endocervicitis that weakens fetal membranes and increases risk of preterm labor and premature rupture of membranes. The neonate can become infected during delivery, resulting in ophthalmia neonatorum. Erythromycin ophthalmic ointment should be administered as a prophylaxis. **Syphilis** may be transmitted placentally, resulting in spontaneous abortion, stillbirth, preterm labor and delivery, and/or congenital syphilis. Transmission rates are 50% to 80% if the mother has untreated primary or secondary syphilis. The fetus is affected after the first trimester, so organs develop normally but all body systems may be affected. Many may appear asymptomatic at birth but exhibit multiple symptoms, such as mucous patches, skin lesions, gumma, and neurological impairment within the first 3 months (early onset) or after 2 years (late onset). Some infants develop meningitis, hydrocephalus, and seizure disorders. Benzathine penicillin G is the drug of choice for treatment of mothers and infants.

- 16 -

Impact of Maternal Diseases on Fetus and Newborn

Herpes and Influenza

Herpes may be transmitted transplacentally (rare) if initial maternal infection occurs during pregnancy and may infect the infant through ascending infection after rupture of the membranes or during delivery. Risk is greatest if the mother is experiencing a primary infection with lesions evident. Caesarean delivery reduces risk of transmission. Placental infection may result in spontaneous abortion. The neonate may develop clusters of vesicles, elevated temperature, poor feeding, seizures, encephalitis, and jaundice. With disseminated infection, neurological impairment or death may occur. Antiviral drugs may be administered to reduce severity. Maternal **influenza** should be treated with antiviral drugs (oseltamivir preferred) within 48 hours of onset and antipyretics to control fever to reduce severity because influenza increases the risk of preterm labor and delivery and stillbirth as well as birth defects of the heart, brain, or spine. The mother is also at increased risk of complications, such as pneumonia. If the mother is immunized, the neonate also has reduced risk for the first 6 months.

Bacterial Vaginosis

Bacterial vaginosis results from imbalance of the normal bacterial flora found in the vagina and is usually characterized by thin white-gray to yellow foul "fishy" smelling discharge and sometimes itching and discomfort although some women may be asymptomatic. The discharge has a pH >4.5. Treatment is typically with oral metronidazole or clindamycin. While antibiotic creams and gels may reduce symptoms, they may be insufficient to protect the pregnancy. Although not considered a sexually transmitted disease, **bacterial vaginosis** is associated with vaginal intercourse. Bacterial vaginosis may result in spontaneous abortion, preterm labor and delivery, premature rupture of membranes, chorioamnionitis, and amnionic fluid infection. The neonate may have a low-birth weight. Maternal treatment reduces the risk of low-birth weight and premature rupture of the membranes, but does not seem to reduce incidence of preterm labor.

Risks and Benefits of Antiviral Therapy on Fetus

Antiviral medications, such as zanamivir or oseltamivir (usually preferred), are routinely administered to pregnant women who have viral infections, such as influenza or herpes. The antivirals are pregnancy class C drugs (indicating safety has not been established during pregnancy), but a number of studies seem to indicate that they do not result in adverse effects on the pregnancy (such as preterm labor or premature rupture of membranes) or on the fetus, as birth defect are within the normal expected range for mothers treated with antiviral medications. Antivirals should be administered within 48 hours of onset of symptoms (such as with influenza) if possible for maximum effect. Dosage may vary depending on the drug and disorder, but treatment is usually for 5 days. Because the adverse effects of viral infections on the mother and the developing fetus are well documented, any risks associated with antiviral therapy are considered acceptable.

Causes of Hemorrhagic Complications During Pregnancy

Hemorrhage during pregnancy puts both fetus and mother at risk of death from hypoxia. Loss of blood predisposes the mother to anemia and infection, and the fetus to premature birth. Placental abruption and uterine rupture are the main causes of hemorrhage resulting in maternal and fetal death. Spontaneous abortion can cause bleeding early in a pregnancy. Ectopic pregnancy is another cause of bleeding early in pregnancy. Placental previa also can result in bleeding early, and can complicate delivery, resulting in the need for a cesarean section. Vasa previa, a condition in which umbilical arteries and veins are in an abnormal position at the opening of the uterus, can result in

- 17 -

vessel rupture during a spontaneous rupture of membranes or an artificial amniotomy and rapid fetus demise from fetal hemorrhage.

Effects of Antiphospholipid Antibody Syndrome and Other Thrombophilias on Pregnancy

Maternal blood is naturally hypercoagulable during pregnancy. **Antiphospholipid antibody syndrome** results when changes occur in platelet and endothelial cell membranes, causing maternal antibodies to form, increasing the risk of clotting. Thrombosis occurs, causing emboli and decreased perfusion of the placenta. Severe preeclampsia, placental abruption, growth retardation, fetal compromise, premature delivery, and fetal death may result. Of the antiphospholipid antibodies, lupus anticoagulant and anticardiolipin antibodies cause the most problems during pregnancies.

Common Blood Disorders of Pregnancy

Megaloblastic Anemia and Physiologic (Iron-Deficient) Anemia of Pregnancy

Folic acid deficiency causes **megaloblastic anemia** in which immature red blood cells enlarge rather than divide, resulting in fewer red blood cells. Because of the need for cell duplication during pregnancy, adequate folic acid is critical, especially because of increased urinary excretion and fetal uptake. Women should receive 0.4mg folic acid daily and, for deficiency, 1mg folic acid and iron supplements (because folic acid deficiency is associated with iron deficiency anemia). During pregnancy, **physiologic (iron-deficient) anemia of pregnancy** occurs because the mother's plasma volume increases by about 50 percent, but red cell mass increases less, so the hematocrit drops from a normal of 38 to 47% to as low as 34%. Because the fetus takes iron, necessary for red blood cell development, from the mother, the mother's iron intake must compensate for this loss. Recommended daily iron supplements include:

- Hematocrit within normal range: 30 mg elemental iron daily.
- Maternal iron deficiency anemia: 60 to 120 mg/daily until hematocrit normalizes, at which point the dose should decrease to 30 mg daily.

Thrombocytopenia

Thrombocytopenia is a platelet count <150,000 mcg/L (normal 150,000 to 450,000 mcg/L). **Gestational thrombocytopenia** often occurs in the third trimester because of hemodilution associated with increased plasma, so some degree of thrombocytopenia is considered within normal parameters and poses little problem. However, thrombocytopenia is also present with hypertension, acute fatty liver, DIC, and pre-eclampsia/eclampsia, so patients need careful monitoring. **Inherited thrombocytopenia** may increase maternal risk of bleeding and may also result in fetal thrombocytopenia if the fetus inherits the condition. Placental infarcts may occur, resulting in fetal demise. **Immune thrombocytopenic purpura** is an autoimmune disorder in which IgG antibodies are directed against platelets, prematurely destroying them. Pregnancy does not increase risk of relapse of exacerbation, but the IgG antibodies may cross the placenta and cause fetal thrombocytopenia, which may result in fetal hemorrhage (especially intracranial). Studies show that fetal platelet count cannot be predicted based on the maternal platelet count.

Hemolytic Anemias

With hemolytic anemias, red blood cells are prematurely destroyed, resulting in mild to severe anemia. Hemolytic anemia may be secondary to other disorders, such as DIC and pre-eclampsia/eclampsia. **Pregnancy-induced hemolytic anemia** is a rare condition in which severe hemolytic anemia develops early in pregnancy and usually persists throughout the pregnancy. The cause is unclear. The fetus may also develop hemolytic anemia, putting it at risk. Some women but

- 18 -

not all, respond to corticosteroid treatment. **Drug-induced hemolytic anemia** results in production of antibodies against red blood cells. Common causes include cephalosporins, NSAIDS, dapsone, and penicillin. The condition is usually mild and resolves after the drug is discontinued. **Bacterial toxin-associated hemolytic anemia** may result from severe pyelonephritis and bacteremia that results in an exotoxin of *Clostridium perfringens* or Group A-β-hemolytic streptococcus. This is the hemolytic anemia that has the most rapid and severe onset during pregnancy.

DIC

Disseminated intravascular coagulation (DIC) is a secondary disorder of pregnancy, which may be triggered by abruptio placentae, uterine rupture, embolism of amniotic fluid, eclampsia, post-partum hemorrhage, shock (hypovolemic), dead fetus, severe infection with sepsis, or saline/missed abortion. DIC triggers both coagulation and hemorrhage through a complex series of events, placing the patient at high risk for death, even with treatment. The onset of DIC may be very rapid.

Symptoms and treatment:

Symptoms	Treatment
Bleeding from surgical, venous puncture, or vaginal sites. Evidence of GI bleeding with distention or bloody diarrhea. Hypotension and acute symptoms of shock. Petechiae and purpura with extensive bleeding into the tissues. Laboratory abnormalities: Prolonged prothrombin and partial prothrombin times. Decreased platelet counts and fragmented RBCs. Decreased fibrinogen.	Identifying and treating underlying cause. Replacement blood products, such as platelets and fresh frozen plasma. Anticoagulation therapy (heparin) to increase clotting time. Cryoprecipitate to increase fibrinogen levels. Coagulation inhibitors and coagulation factors.

Fetal Risks from Maternal Type I and Type II Diabetes

Preexisting maternal diabetes, whether type I or II, increases the risk of congenital abnormalities of the fetus. Poor maternal glycemic control is a large factor causing defects at a rate that is 3 to 4 times more frequent than normal pregnancies. Heart defects and neural tube defects occur and frequently defects are more severe and numerous in these fetuses. Fetal growth and metabolism is affected and fetal acidosis can occur. The rate of fetal demise is increased 2.5-fold in diabetic pregnancies with miscarriages and stillbirths more common. Large infants can cause the need for cesarean births and may be at risk for hypoglycemia after birth. Maternal vascular complications of diabetes increase the risk of fetal growth retardation and increase the risk of pregnancy-induced hypertension, which further compromises blood flow to the fetus. Polycythemia of the infant caused by maternal hyperglycemia, hyperinsulinemia, and hyperketonemia increases the occurrence of hyperbilirubinemia after birth. These infants also frequently have low serum calcium and magnesium levels.

Fetal Risks from Gestational Diabetes

Gestational diabetes is diabetes that is caused by and first detected during pregnancy. When it occurs in the first trimester there is a high a risk for congenital abnormalities if maternal glycemic control is poor. For women with **gestational diabetes** under good glycemic control, the risk of fetal death is no higher than a normal pregnancy. However, perinatal problems such as postmaturity, asphyxia, metabolic abnormalities, hypoglycemia, and respiratory distress syndrome occur more often in these infants. Macrosomia occurs even with good glycemic control and delivery trauma is more likely with vaginal births. Shoulder dystocia is the most common birth injury. The rate of cesarean section deliveries is higher because of macrosomia.

Impact of Maternal Cardiac Disease on Pregnancy

Pregnancy puts a strain on the woman's cardiovascular system that is worsened by the presence of **cardiac disease**. The most common is rheumatic heart disease. A pregnant woman may also have a congenital heart defect, arrhythmia, or another cardiomyopathy present. Each of these maternal cardiac problems has their own risk of maternal/fetal morbidity and mortality, but most pregnancies have a good outcome. A maternal congenital heart defect may be passed on to the fetus. Abnormal fetal cardiac development can occur if maternal cardiac output is decreased during the time the heart is forming. Decreased output may result in decreased nourishment to the fetus and growth retardation, and decreased reserves can occur in the fetus. Mothers who do well during pregnancy may be severely stressed by labor and delivery. The risk for a myocardial infarction increases during this time.

Fetal Risks from Maternal Hypothyroidism and Hyperthyroidism

Maternal hypothyroidism threatens the development of the fetal brain and spinal cord. T4 is needed for proper development and the fetus is not capable of T4 production during the critical period of growth. Decreased mental capacity or fetal death can occur. **Hyperthyroidism** is difficult to detect since symptoms mimic normal pregnancy problems. The pregnant woman may have temporary hyperthyroidism in early pregnancy but levels should return to normal by the beginning of the second trimester. Continued high levels can cause thyroid crisis and result in fetal death or premature birth.

Common Pulmonary Problems During Pregnancy

Most pregnant women develop mild shortness of breath at rest and with light exercise during pregnancy. About 30% of pregnant women develop rhinitis with nasal congestion because of hormonal changes during pregnancy. Sleep apnea can occur, especially when obesity or rhinitis is also present. The new onset of snoring in the pregnant mother should be investigated since the coexistence of hypertension or preeclampsia with snoring is associated with intrauterine growth retardation and decreased Apgar scores. Thromboembolic disease and amniotic fluid embolism are the most common causes of unexpected maternal deaths during labor and delivery.

Pregnancy Risks with Maternal Asthma

The most common pulmonary disease seen in pregnant women is **asthma**. About 33% of women with asthma find that symptoms get worse during pregnancy; the rest find that symptoms improve or remain the same as before pregnancy. Symptoms often worsen during weeks 24 to 36, after which they tend to improve. Pregnancy complications that can occur when asthma is present include hyperemesis, preeclampsia, vaginal bleeding, infections, gestational diabetes, premature labor or rupture of membranes, and an extended recovery period after birth. The fetus is not at increased risk when the asthma is well controlled but exacerbations can result in decreased oxygen to the fetus, growth retardation, oligohydramnios, distress causing meconium-staining, premature delivery, and fetal distress resulting in death.

Pregnancy Risks with Maternal Pneumonia

Pneumonia is the third leading cause of maternal deaths in the United States. When it occurs during pregnancy it is more severe in nature and pregnant women have less physical tolerance for the disease. It occurs more among poor pregnant women, in older pregnant women, and in those with other medical problems or using illegal drugs, or who are immunodeficient. Complications to the mother include preterm labor, pulmonary complications such as emphysema, pneumothorax, or respiratory failure, and atrial fibrillation or pericardial tamponade. The fetus can be severely stressed by maternal hypoxemia, and growth retardation or fetal death can occur. Premature birth and its complications can also threaten the baby.

Causes of Acute Pulmonary Edema During Pregnancy

Acute pulmonary edema during pregnancy can be caused by heart failure, tocolytic drugs given to prevent premature labor, or a combination of the two. Sepsis is frequently involved as well. Rapid fluid therapy can predispose the woman to pulmonary edema. Woman who receive tocolytics for more than 48 hours or combined with magnesium sulfate infusion, or who have diabetes, preeclampsia, infections, cardiac problems, blood transfusions, or multiple pregnancy are at highest risk for **pulmonary edema**. Maternal hypoxemia deprives the fetus of adequate oxygen supply and can result in fetal distress, death, or premature birth.

Effects of Maternal Trauma on Fetus

Maternal trauma can occur at anytime during the pregnancy. Motor vehicle accidents are the leading cause of trauma to the pregnant woman. Maternal falls and trauma to the abdomen from domestic abuse are other common causes. Trauma to the abdomen by blunt force can result in abruptio placentae, placental injury, injury to the fetus, or uterine rupture causing fetal death by hemorrhage and hypoxia. Maternal hemorrhage and shock from traumatic injuries can result in both fetal and maternal death from hypoxia. Any trauma that compromises respiration will also cause hypoxia to the mother-fetal unit. Neurological trauma that results in shock, hemorrhage, or damage to the brain will also compromise the fetus when maternal vital functions deteriorate.

Hyperemesis Gravidarum

Hyperemesis gravidarum is a persistent nausea and vomiting that occurs during pregnancy. While mild to moderate nausea and vomiting during weeks 4 through 16 are common among pregnant women, vomiting that is severe enough to cause dehydration, electrolyte and acid-base imbalances, and weight loss threatens both mother and fetus. Hospitalization may be required to stabilize the mother. Estrogens and human chorionic gonadotropin (hCG) are thought to be involved but the exact cause of nausea and vomiting during pregnancy is not well understood. It occurs more often with female fetuses. Complications can include vitamin K and thiamine deficiencies, Mallory-Weiss tears, rupture of the esophagus, pneumothorax, pneumomediastinum, and maternal renal failure.

Kidney and Urinary Tract Diseases During Pregnancy

Pregnancy increases the incidence of **pyelonephritis** and can cause **chronic renal disease** to get worse. The ureters and renal calyces dilate and this can cause bacteria to ascend from the lower tract to the upper, causing kidney infection. Some women have bacteria in the urine in early

- 21 -

pregnancy without symptoms of infection. This is treated to prevent a bladder or kidney infection from developing. Pyelonephritis can escalate to septic shock and may cause cerebral palsy in premature infants. Women with chronic kidney disease must have renal function and the degree of hypertension evaluated prior to becoming pregnant. Even if function is good and hypertension is absent or minimal, there may be an increased incidence of preeclampsia, fetal growth retardation, and prematurity.

Impact of Pregnancy on Epilepsy

Headaches are the most common neurological condition in pregnancy and **epilepsy** is the second most common. Seizures increase in frequency in about 35% of women with epilepsy. This is often due to a lower seizure threshold and subtherapeutic levels of anticonvulsants because of pregnancy-induced alterations in the metabolism of anticonvulsant drugs. Seizure thresholds can be lower when the woman loses sleep, or is stressed by pain during labor. Many anticonvulsant drugs cause birth defects, so the drug chosen should be one with less risk of defects. About 10% of the children born to women with epilepsy will develop epilepsy later in life.

Rhesus and ABO Incompatibility

Both Rhesus and ABO incompatibility involve a mother and fetus with different blood types. If fetal blood escapes into maternal circulation and the mother is D- or has blood type O, she will make antibodies if the fetal blood is D+, or type A or B. These antibodies can then threaten subsequent pregnancies if the fetus has D+ or type A or B blood. The antibodies cause hemolysis of the fetal red blood cells, which results in anemia. If the anemia is severe, erythroblastosis fetalis can occur and the fetus may die without an intrauterine blood transfusion. As a neonate, hyperbilirubinemia can occur with the threat of kernicterus, and cause CNS damage and cerebral palsy if bilirubin levels are high. Infant deaths occur much less frequently in the United States since the advent of the use of D-immunoglobulin.

Normal AFI, Oligohydramnios, and Polyhydramnios

The **amniotic fluid index** (AFI) is determined by measuring the biggest pockets of amniotic fluid in all four of the uterine quadrants and adding the measurements together. The **normal index** is from 5 to 24 cm, depending on which week of gestation the measurements are taken. Amniotic fluid volume increases during pregnancy to 1,000 mL by 36 weeks of gestation, then slowly decreases over the next 4 weeks. **Oligohydramnios** is defined by an AFI of 5 cm or less. It is linked with fetal urinary tract anomalies. The fetus is threatened by the risk of amnion adhesions that can cause amputation of body parts and pressure that can cause deformities of the musculoskeletal system, especially club foot. Cord compression and fetal distress can occur during labor and delivery. **Polyhydramnios** is defined by an AFI over 24 cm. It can occur acutely or over time. One-third of these cases are associated with fetal anomalies of the CNS or GI systems, maternal diabetes, or multifetal gestation. More severe polyhydramnios increases the risk of perinatal death.

Acute Fatty Liver of Pregnancy

Acute fatty liver of pregnancy (**AFLP**) (the most common cause of liver failure during pregnancy) is characterized by micro-vesicular fat deposits throughout the liver that crowd out hepatocytes and interfere with liver function. AFLP, which is associated with genetic mutations, occurs in the third trimester or postpartal period. Women may exhibit nausea and vomiting, upper GI hemorrhage, coagulopathy, hypoglycemia, pancreatitis, hypoglycemia, hepatic encephalopathy (with confusion and altered mental status), hypertension, jaundice, general malaise, and renal and hepatic failure. Neonates may exhibit fatty acid oxidation defects that affect multiple body systems:

- 22 -

cardiomyopathy, liver failure, myopathy, neuropathy, and hypoglycemia (nonketotic). Some may die *in utero* and 15% after birth. The key to treatment of AFLP is immediate delivery of the fetus through labor induction or Caesarean (although coagulopathy may pose risks). Supportive care may include IV fluids, blood products, coagulation factors, and/or plasma exchange or plasmapheresis with continuous renal replacement therapy. Some women may require liver transplantation.

Systemic Lupus Erythematosus

Systemic lupus erythematosus (**SLE**), a systemic reaction to collagen or connective tissue in the body, is believed triggered by an antibody-antigen immune response to an environmental agent, resulting in widespread damage of vessels and organs, primarily in females. Symptoms may include: malar and discoid rash; photosensitivity; oral ulcers; arthritis; serositis; and renal (proteinuria/nephritis), neurological (seizures, psychosis), and immunological disorders. Pregnant women with SLE have high rates of hypertension (up to 30%) and preeclampsia, especially with lupus nephritis, so they may need to continue immunosuppressive drugs during pregnancy. Women must be monitored carefully during pregnancy for flare-ups of SLE. Impaired circulation to the fetus may result from maternal decidual vasculopathy with placental infarction. Fetal risks include preterm delivery, fetal growth restriction, spontaneous abortion, and stillbirths. The newborn may inherit neonatal lupus, with symptoms appearing up to 4 weeks after birth. Indications include congenital heart block, autoimmune hemolysis, thrombocytopenia, and lupus dermatitis.

Cholelithiasis and Cholecystitis

Pregnancy increases the risk of a woman developing cholelithiasis and cholecystitis because of increased levels of estrogen and increased biliary sludge (forerunner to gallstones). Symptoms occur when stones block the bile duct and may include RUQ pain, nausea, vomiting, low-grade fever, and mildly elevated white blood cell count. Some may have clay-colored stools and jaundice. Medical management has been most common in the first and third trimesters and surgical repair in the second trimester (when it is safest); however, early cholecystitis often recurs later in the pregnancy, increasing the risk of pre-term delivery and making surgery more difficult because of the size of the uterus, so some authorities advise against conservative treatment. Surgical procedures include laparoscopic cholecystectomy and endoscopic retrograde cholangiopancreatography for stones in the common bile duct. The fetus is usually unimpaired if the blockage is resolved.

Impact of Maternal Obesity and Age on Pregnancy

The numbers of mothers who are obese or older than 35 years of age are increasing. Both conditions increase the risk of morbidity and mortality for mother and fetus. Complications of pregnancy are more numerous in these two groups and include a higher risk of ischemic events, preeclampsia, gestational diabetes, stillbirth, and premature births. Labor and delivery can be complicated by macrosomia, failure to progress, cesarean section deliveries, problems with anesthetics, and postpartum hemorrhages. Infection and wound dehiscence are more common. Fetal anomalies such as spina bifida and ventral wall defects, distress during labor and delivery, and postnatal neonatal problems occur at a higher rate because of the complications rather than the obesity and age.

Guidelines for Pregnancy Post-Bariatric Surgery

Patients are usually advised to avoid pregnancy for at least 18 months **post-bariatric surgery** to give the patient time to stabilize weight loss. Pregnancy soon after surgery may result in small-for-gestational age neonates. The primary concern with pregnancy post-bariatric surgery is the maternal nutritional status because many patients have deficiencies of protein, iron, and calcium as well as vitamin deficiencies (especially vitamins B12 and D), and their caloric intake may be 500 to 1000 kcal/day, which is not sufficient to support pregnancy. Thus, patient's nutritional status should be monitored at least every trimester. The patient may need to eat several small nutritious meals daily. Additionally, absorption of medications may be impaired, and symptoms of pregnancy (nausea, vomiting, discomfort) may mimic those of post-bariatric complications, so careful evaluation is necessary. Patients still overweight are at increased risk of hypertension and gestational diabetes. Labor and delivery should progress normally in post-bariatric patients.

Pregnancy Risks Affecting the Fetus and Newborn

Maternal Factors That Impact Fetus and Neonate

Stress, Weight, Health Habits, and Exercise

Many **maternal factors** have an impact on the fetus and newborn:

- **Stress**: Effects the neurodevelopment of the fetus, resulting in behavioral and neurological impairments as the child grows. The fetus exposed to maternal stress has less variability in fetal heart rate. If the mother is depressed, the fetus tends to be more active; and if anxious, less active.
- **Weight**: Inadequate weight gain during pregnancy can result in low-birth weight, preterm labor, and increased mortality and morbidity. Excess weight can result in macrosomia, prolonged labor, Caesarean delivery, birth trauma, and asphyxia.
- **Health habits**: Smoking can result in low birth rate, spontaneous abortion, placental abruption, preterm birth and developmental problems in the infant. Alcohol is a teratogen and can lead to fetal alcohol syndrome with cognitive and physical impairment and skeletal and organ malformations.
- **Exercise**: Can improve circulation, improve sleep, elevate mood, decrease duration of labor, aand prevent excess weight gain. However, it can also impair oxygenation to the fetus and increase risk of maternal falls.

Maternal Alcohol Ingestion During Pregnancy

Maternal ingestion of alcohol during pregnancy can cause **fetal alcohol syndrome**. The level of ingestion needed to cause defects has not been determined. Fetal alcohol syndrome is characterized physically by a distinctive facies with a flat midface, short palpebral fissures, epicanthal folds, a hypoplastic philtrum, and a thin upper lip. Heart or joint deformities may be present. The infant may fail to thrive, be irritable during early childhood, and have growth and developmental deficits. Mental capacity varies, and attention deficit hyperactivity disorder, cerebral palsy, epilepsy, learning problems, and poor coordination can occur in these children.

Smoking During Pregnancy

The risk of negative effects on the fetus increases with the amount that the pregnant woman **smokes** and during which part of the pregnancy she smokes. Smoking has been shown to result in retardation of fetal growth, resulting in low birthweight. Smoking during the first trimester can also result in cardiac or other defects. The risk of placental problems such as placenta previa and abruptio placenta is doubled. Premature rupture of membranes, causing premature birth, also occurs as a result of smoking. The neonate may suffer withdrawal after birth with symptoms of jitteriness and difficulty soothing. The risk of sudden infant death syndrome (SIDS) is tripled in these neonates.

Maternal Cocaine Use

Cocaine acts as a vasoconstrictor. Its hypertensive effects affect maternal and fetal circulation. There is a 4-fold increased risk of abruptio placenta and increased risk of fetal demise. Intrauterine growth restriction can occur. Possible fetal abnormalities include skull and facial defects, microcephaly and other brain anomalies, cutis aplasia, ileal atresia, cardiac anomalies, genitourinary tract anomalies, and visceral infarction. Developmental and cognitive deficiencies also occur. The neonate may suffer withdrawal symptoms. These women may also take other illicit drugs, drink alcohol, and smoke. Nutritional deficiencies and general poor health is common and adds to the overall risk of a poor pregnancy outcome.

Pica

Pica is the craving for unusual or nonfood items. The most common nonfood items eaten by pregnant women are laundry starch, sourdough, and ice. Clay or dirt is also eaten. It is thought to be an unusual maternal physiological reaction to the presence of *iron deficiency anemia* but not all women with pica are anemic. If the woman eats too much of these nonfood items, iron deficiency and other nutritional deficiencies will develop. Women with pica have a risk that is twice as high as normal of preterm delivery earlier than 35 weeks.

Prevalence of Anxiety Disorders Amongst Pregnant Women

Pregnancy-specific anxiety is high in pregnant women, especially in the first and third trimesters, but the rates of **anxiety disorders**, such as depression, are similar to those of non-pregnant women. Approximately 10-13% of pregnant women suffer from depression. Rates of OCD and generalized anxiety disorder show a slight increase during pregnancy, and panic attacks may start or worsen. Anxiety increases perceptions of pain by triggering release of catecholamines, which increase pelvic pain stimuli transmitted to the CNS and may be a major factor in labor pain. Additionally, anxiety increases muscle tension, decreasing the effectiveness of uterine contractions and prolonging labor. The increased pain further increases anxiety. Treatment to reduce anxiety includes providing analgesia to reduce pain, keeping the woman informed with accurate information about progress, and ensuring comfort measures, such as relaxation exercises, massage, breathing techniques, and quiet, calm environment.

Effects of Anti-Anxiety Medications on Fetus and Newborn

Commonly used medications to treat anxiety may pose risks to the fetus and newborn, so risks and benefits should be discussed with the physician. Typical medications include:

- **Benzodiazepines** (alprazolam, lorazepam, diazepam, clonazepam): Study results have been inconsistent in regards to whether benzodiazepines cause birth defect or development/behavior problems, but the neonate may have withdrawal symptoms, such as dyspnea, tremors, jitters, excessive crying, and difficulty sleeping. Combining benzodiazepines with diphenhydramine may result in increased rate of stillbirths.
- **Buspirone**: Little data regarding pregnancy is available for this drug, but it is classified as a Class B drug.

- **SSRIs** (fluoxetine, sertraline, citalopram, paroxetine, escitalopram): May cause persistent pulmonary hypertension of the newborn if taken during the last 50% of the pregnancy. Paroxetine (Paxil®) may result in congenital heart disease. Withdrawal symptoms in neonate may occur within 2 days of delivery and may be similar to those of benzodiazepines.
- **SNRIs** (venlaxafine, duloxetine): Similar to SSRIs although withdrawal symptoms are less pronounced.

Alternate Treatments for Anxiety and Depression During Pregnancy

Many pregnant women choose to avoid medications for anxiety and depression out of concern for possible adverse effects on the fetus, but these untreated disorders pose risks as well, so **alternate treatments** should be provided:

- **Bright light therapy**: Patient sits in front of light box (10,000 lux) for 30 minutes in AM to treat depression.
- **Cognitive behavioral therapy**: Helps the patient to control thought patterns and control depression and anxiety disorders.
- **Group therapy**: Talking with others with similar anxiety provides emotional support.
- **Relaxation exercises/Visualization**: Helps the patient to control emotional response and to reduce anxiety.
- **Support/Reassurance**: Anticipating questions and providing clear and honest information about what to expect during pregnancy and the patient's progress can help to allay fears and reduce anxiety.
- **Exercise**: Physical exercise, such as daily walks, can help to increase release of endorphins and increase feeling of wellbeing.

Impact of Drugs on Fetus and Newborn

Heroin and Methadone

Heroin: Users may experience poor nutrition, iron deficiency anemia, and preeclampsia-eclampsia, all negatively affecting the fetus. Premature birth, early placental separation, and breech presentation are common. If the mother tries to stop using heroin, she may go into withdrawal, which can trigger premature labor, spontaneous abortion, or stillbirth. While neonates may exhibit jitteriness, fever, poor feeding, and vomiting after birth, the symptoms are usually transient.

Methadone: Often administered to pregnant women to decrease dangers associated with heroin, such as fluctuating levels of drug and exposure to hepatitis and HIV from sharing of needles. Exposure to methadone may result in miscarriage, stillbirth, intrauterine growth restriction, fetal distress, and low birth rate although symptoms are usually less severe than with heroin. Sudden withdrawal from methadone may cause preterm labor or death of the fetus, so methadone should be monitored carefully.

Marijuana and Buprenorphine Products

While no teratogenic effects of marijuana have been demonstrated, the active component (THC) of **marijuana** passes through the placenta and stays in the fetus for up to a month, and carbon monoxide levels are 5 times higher than with cigarettes. The fetus may exhibit intrauterine growth restriction and the neonate negative neurological signs, such as tremors, hyperirritability, and photosensitivity. Additionally, infants may show some degree of cognitive and language impairment for 4 years. Women who use marijuana during pregnancy may also engage in other high-risk

- 26 -

activities that can endanger the fetus. **Buprenorphine products** (Suboxone® and Subutex®) are used during pregnancy to prevent opioid withdrawal, which can lead to spontaneous abortion and preterm labor. Suboxone® contains naloxone, which is dangerous to the fetus because it can lead to withdrawal if the drug is abused, so pregnant women are given Subutex®. Buprenorphine causes neonatal abstinence syndrome, but less severely than other opioids.

Prescription and Over-the-Counter Medications

Prescription and over-the-counter drugs vary in danger to the fetus and newborn. Drugs submitted to the FDA before June 30, 2015 use the A-D, X system to indicate fetal risk with A safe, B probably safe, C and D some risk, and X unsafe. Drugs submitted later have a narrative explanation of risk. Drugs that pose a particular risk to the fetus and are frequently abused are opioids, stimulants, barbiturates, and benzodiazepines. Drugs classified as *A* include vitamins and thyroid medications. Even *B* drugs should be taken only if necessary. Many common drugs may pose some risk of birth defects. SSRIs may cause persistent pulmonary hypertension of the newborn if taken during the last 50% of the pregnancy. Paroxetine (Paxil®) may result in fetal heart defects. MAOIs may result in intrauterine growth restriction. Some medications taken for hypertension (ACE inhibitors and ARBs) should be avoided. Warfarin use during pregnancy may result in spontaneous abortion, fetal hemorrhage, and risk of multiple birth defects. Even "safe" OTC drugs, such as acetaminophen, may increase risk of ADHD during childhood.

Impact of Environmental Toxins and Elements on Fetus and Newborn

Toxic waste products to which the pregnant woman are exposed can enter the bloodstream and cross the placenta, affecting fetal development or resulting in delayed health disorders, such as ADHD, hypertension, heart disease, and cancer as the child grows. Toxins that are of particular concern to the developing fetus and neonate include:

- **Dioxins and furans**: Neonate has increased risk of developmental disorders and cancer.
- **Polychlorinated biphenyls** (PCBs): Neonates with low birth weight, small head circumference, and neurological impairment, including motor and cognitive abilities.
- **Mercury**: Neurological damage to the developing fetus, resulting in small head circumference, mental retardation, blindness, seizures, and cerebral palsy.
- **Lead**: Spontaneous abortion, preterm delivery, low birth rate, damage to neurological system (including the brain) and kidney. Later development of learning and behavioral problems.
- **Bisphenol A** (BPA): May affect fetal brain development.

Prevalence of Intimate Partner Violence Amongst Pregnant Women

Up to 25% of women in the United States have suffered intimate partner violence (**IPV**), and 45% of women who are victims of IPV continue to be abused during pregnancy, and in some cases violence starts with pregnancy or escalates, especially if the partner resents the pregnancy. All pregnant women should be routinely screened for IPV by asking directly about abuse when the partner is absent as women may be rightfully fearful. The risk to the fetus is high, especially if the partner targets the abdomen as this can cause placental injury and placental abruption. IPV during pregnancy is associated with greater risk of low-birth weight, preterm birth, and neonatal mortality. Risk factors for IPV during pregnancy include recent immigrants (especially from cultures in which violence toward women is common), history of child abuse, prior IPV, substance abuse, history of depression/suicide attempts, young age (<24), low education, and unplanned pregnancy. In >50% of cases of IPV, the children are also at risk of abuse.

- 27 -

Classic Signs and Symptoms of Intimate Partner Violence

Injuries consistent with intimate partner violence/abuse:

Characteristic injuries	Ruptured eardrum. Rectal/genital injury—burns, bites, trauma. Scrapes and bruises about the neck, face, head, trunk, arms. Cuts, bruises, and fractures of the face. Pregnant women often have injuries in multiple body areas, especially the abdomen, breasts, and genitalia.
Patterns of injuries	Bathing suit pattern—injuries on parts of body that are usually covered with clothing as the perpetrator abuses but hides evidence of abuse. Head and neck injuries (50%).
Abusive injuries (rarely attributable to accidents)	Bites, bruises, rope and cigarette burns, welts in the outline of weapons (belt marks). Bilateral injuries of arms/legs.
Defensive injuries	Back of the body injury from being attacked while crouched on the floor face down. Soles of the feet from kicking at perpetrator. Ulnar aspect of hand or palm from blocking blows.

Assessment for and Response to Domestic/Dating Violence

Assessment for **intimate partner violence** should be done for all patients, regardless of background, lifestyle, or signs of abuse. The nurse should be informed about IPV and aware or risk factors, typical injuries, and danger signs. The interview should be conducted in private (or with children <3 years old). The office, bathrooms, and examining rooms should have information about IPV posted prominently. Brochures and information should be available to give to patients. Patients may present with a variety of physical complaints, such as headache, pain, palpitations, numbness, or pelvic pain. They are often depressed and may appear suicidal and may be isolated from friends and family. Victims of IPV often exhibit fear of perpetrator (such as a parent, spouse, boyfriend, or girlfriend) and may report injury inconsistent with symptoms. If a patient admits to injuries from IPV, the first question should be, "Is the person who hurt you here?" because security may need to be called. It's important to remain supportive and nonjudgmental and to provide information and assistance.

- 28 -

Fetal Assessment

Antepartum Assessment

Comprehensive Prenatal Diagnostic Evaluation

Women who are at high risk of having a fetus with congenital problem should be offered a **comprehensive diagnostic evaluation**. This includes women older than 35 years of age and women older than 32 years of age who have a twin pregnancy. Any abnormality seen during ultrasound should be investigated further. A positive family history of congenital anomalies, genetic disorders, or chromosomal abnormalities should prompt evaluation and counseling when appropriate. Evaluation is done using ultrasound, chorionic villus sampling, amniocentesis, and maternal and fetal blood sampling. The cervical or vaginal fluid can be tested for biochemical markers.

Baseline Health Information Gathered at Initial Prenatal Visit

Baseline health information is collected to determine the risks to the pregnancy. Information to be gathered includes a thorough health history that includes the woman's reproductive history and a family health history. Exposure to possible teratogens should be assessed. A comprehensive physical exam is performed next, with emphasis on any health finding that could affect the pregnancy. Uterine size and fundal height is determined. Blood is collected for lab screening tests and tests appropriate to any medical condition present at the time. The fetus should be evaluated by listening for the fetal heart rate (FHR) if appropriate to the gestational age. Fetal activity, ultrasound imaging, and a biophysical profile may be obtained.

Ultrasound

Ultrasound uses high-frequency sound waves that are intermittent to view the fetus, placenta, uterus, and adnexa. It is the procedure used most commonly on pregnant women. **Ultrasound** is able to confirm the presence of a gestational sac and can detect multiple sacs and fetuses. The crown-rump length of the fetus helps to determine the approximate gestational age to within a week. Fetal heart motion can be seen and the sex can be determined. Placental location, amniotic fluid volume, and fetal lie can be determined. Many fetal anomalies have been found during a routine ultrasound screening. Ultrasound is also used to guide other procedures such as percutaneous umbilical cord blood sampling.

Three-Dimensional Ultrasonography During Pregnancy

Three-dimensional ultrasonography provides a superior picture of the fetal body. The portion of the body that is to be examined must be free-floating in the amniotic fluid and not crowded to show the best. It can take extra time and skill to get a usable image. It is most often used to view the extremities, ears, or face. Three-dimensional ultrasonography can confirm fetal anomalies and give details not seen on two-dimensional ultrasound. American College of Obstetricians and Gynecologists (ACOG) recommends that it be used only when medically indicated and not just for the purpose of taking a picture of the fetal face.

CVS

Chorionic villus sampling (CVS) is performed by inserting a catheter into the uterus to obtain placental villi for testing. The tissue may also be obtained through the abdominal wall if needed to

- 29 -

safely reach the placenta. Chromosomal, DNA, and enzymatic analysis is done on the tissue. This test is best performed at 10 to 13 weeks of gestation. This test provides results during early pregnancy to either reassure parents or to provide information needed to decide whether to continue the pregnancy. There is a small risk of fetal injury resulting in death during the procedure.

Fetal Growth Assessment

The uterine fundus can be palpated above the symphysis pubis by about 10 to 12 weeks gestation, and fundal height can be used to estimate **duration of gestation and fetal growth**. Starting at about week 16 gestation and lasting until week 36, the fundal height (from top of symphysis pubis to top of fundus) measured in centimeters usually conforms with the weeks of gestation, so 18 cm is consistent with 18 weeks gestation in a pregnancy with a normal single fetus. At 20 weeks (20 cm), the fundus is usually at the umbilicus. After 36 weeks, the fundal height may increase slowly or decrease as the head engages in preparation for delivery. Ultrasound may also be utilized to assess fetal growth. Crown to rump length is measured during the first trimester, but during the second and third trimester several measurements are used, including biparietal diameter, femur length, and abdominal circumference.

SGA

Small for gestational age (SGA) infants are those whose weight places them below the 10th percentile for their gestational age. SGA is also called dysmaturity. SGA babies commonly aspirate meconium, and have a low APGAR score, asphyxia, hypoglycemia, and polycythemia. Common causes of SGA include:

- Multiple gestations (twins, triplets, quadruplets).
- Constitutional SGA because both parents are small.
- Many genetic defects, such as trisomy 18 (Edwards syndrome), Down syndrome, and Turner syndrome.
- Placental malfunction or misplacement (inadequate fetal nutrition from reduced blood flow, sepsis, placenta previa, or abruptio placentae).
- Maternal disease (pre-eclampsia; high blood pressure; malnutrition; advanced diabetes mellitus; chronic kidney, heart, or respiratory disease; and anemia).
- Infections such as cytomegalovirus, toxoplasmosis, and rubella.
- Maternal tobacco, illegal drug, or alcohol use during pregnancy.
- Birth defects.

FGR/IUGR

When a fetus does not fulfill his or her growth potential for any reason, the diagnosis is **fetal/intrauterine growth restriction (FGR/IUGR)**. Prenatal ultrasound is used to diagnose FGR/IUGR, which is associated with oligohydramnios (decreased amniotic fluid) and pre-eclampsia

Copyright © Mometrix Media. You have been licensed one copy of this document for personal use only. Any other reproduction or redistribution is strictly prohibited. All rights reserved.

(pregnancy-induced hypertension and proteinuria). FGR/IUGR is classified as symmetric or asymmetric, based on the size of the newborn's head:

Symmetric IUGR	Asymmetric IUGR
Both head and body are small (growth-restricted). Occurs early in pregnancy. Common causes are chromosomal abnormalities and infections.	Large head in proportion to the body; the head is spared. The head is normal in size for gestational age, while the body is growth-restricted. Occurs late in pregnancy. Common causes include placental insufficiency and preeclampsia.

LGA

Large for gestational age (LGA) infants are those whose weight places them above the 90th percentile for their gestational age. The main pathologic cause for LGA is maternal diabetes (either gestational diabetes or diabetes mellitus). Infants exposed to elevated levels of glucose produce elevated amounts of insulin, which has an anabolic effect on the developing fetus, causing macrosomia (large body). Poor control of diabetes during pregnancy generally results in a larger infant with these common health problems:

- Delivery complications (shoulder dystocia, clavicle fracture, prolonged vaginal exit requiring use of forceps or Caesarian section, and perinatal asphyxia).
- Abnormal blood test results (hypoglycemia developing within 1-2 hours of birth, hyperbilirubinemia, hypocalcemia, hypomagnesemia, hyperviscosity [thickened blood] secondary to polycythemia [elevated platelets]).
- Jaundice.
- Feeding intolerance.
- Lethargy.
- Respiratory distress.
- Birth defects.

Amniocentesis

Amniocentesis is the insertion of a 20 to 22 gauge spinal needle through the abdominal wall into the amniotic sac to obtain amniotic fluid for analysis. Ultrasound is used to guide the procedure to avoid injuring the fetus, umbilical cord, or placenta. When done before 14 weeks, the sample can only contain 1 mL for each week of gestation. Early **amniocentesis** is much more difficult and carries a higher risk of fetal death, membrane rupture, and foot deformities such as club feet due to the withdrawal of fluid. Most amniocentesis procedures are done at 14 to 20 weeks of gestation for these reasons. The fluid is cultured and genetic studies can be done. Biochemical disorders, CNS anomalies, ventral wall defects, and other disorders can be diagnosed in this way. Complications of the procedure include injury to the fetus, short-term vaginal bleeding, leakage of amniotic fluid, or infection.

PUBS

Percutaneous umbilical cord blood sampling (PUBS, also called cordocentesis) obtains fetal blood cells. A 22-gauge spinal needle is inserted into the umbilical vein at or very near the place where it joins the placenta while using ultrasound to guide placement. Fetal blood is collected and used to assess red cell and platelet status. Fetal blood cells are also used for genetic analysis with

- 31 -

karyotyping available within 24 to 48 hours. Immunological, hematological, and metabolic studies can be done. The fetal acid-base balance can also be determined. Complications of the procedure include fetal injury or death, fetal bradycardia, amniotic fluid loss, vaginal bleeding, infections, or bleeding into the cord or from the fetus into the mother's circulation. The procedure may be done to verify results from other tests.

Fetal Movement Counting

Fetal movements signify fetal well-being. It is an easy, noninvasive way for the mother to monitor her fetus. There is no hard and fast rule as to the ideal number of **fetal movements** within a specific timeframe. However, guidance exists as to the reassuring number. The **count** is considered reassuring if there are 10 movements within 2 hours. A baseline count should be done and succeeding counts can be measured against that number instead. Pregnancies that are high risk should prompt the health care provider to instruct the woman to monitor fetal movements up to 3 times a week after 26 weeks if indicated. Others can wait until 32 weeks to monitor movements. The woman should notify the physician if movements decrease or cease. This can occur because of medications, fetal sleep periods, time of day, placental position, smoking, glucose intake, and decreased space in the uterus as pregnancy progresses. It may also be due to fetal distress or demise.

Fetal Fibronectin

Fetal fibronectin is a glycoprotein produced by many different fetal cells. It can be detected in maternal blood, amniotic fluid, and cervicovaginal secretions. It is involved in implantation, placental adhesion, and cervical changes prior to the onset of labor. Its presence in cervicovaginal secretions is predictive of premature labor within 1 to 2 weeks. Women in preterm labor with intact membranes who do not have **fetal fibronectin** in the cervix or vaginal secretions usually do not go on to deliver prematurely. This knowledge guides obstetrical care.

The mother is cautioned not to have intercourse or douche within 24 hours of the test. Cervical examination must not be done in the previous 24 hours either. A swab is used to obtain a sampling of the cervicovaginal secretions that is free of maternal blood and amnionic fluid. The presence of fibronectin in the secretions predicts preterm labor about 30% of the time. A negative test is the most accurate and is used to avoid tocolytics and other measures to arrest premature labor.

Biophysical Profile

The biophysical profile evaluates fetal status by using electronic monitoring and ultrasonography. It assesses muscle tone, movement, breathing, and reactivity of the FHR. Amniotic fluid volume is also assessed. Nonstress testing is also included. A score of 0 or 2 is given for each item, with a perfect score being 10. A total score of 0 or 2 is abnormal and indicates the likely need for immediate delivery. A score of 4 warns of the possible need for delivery depending on gestational age. A score of 6 signals the need for delivery of the term infant or re-testing the next day for the premature infant.

Biophysical Profile and Modified Biophysical Profile

A biophysical profile assesses the fetal muscle tone, breathing, movements, reactivity of the FHR, and amniotic fluid volume. The **modified biophysical profile** assesses only the reactivity of the FHR and amniotic fluid volume. The amniotic fluid volume should be greater than 5 and the reactivity parameters of the nonstress test are used (2 increases of the FHR to at least 15 beats per minute above the baseline lasting for 15 seconds, with or without noted movements, within 20

- 32 -

minutes of each other). This abbreviated test may be done to monitor the fetal status more easily and quickly since it indicates fetal status as well as more involved tests.

Nonstress Test

Nonstress testing involves electronic monitoring of the FHR while the mother monitors fetal movement. She notifies the nurse of movement and the FHR is examined to see if there is a normal corresponding transient rise in heart rate. If the heart rate does not rise it can signify fetal distress. Monitoring is done for 20 to 40 minutes. The normal goal is two incidences of an increase in FHR to at least 15 beats per minute above the baseline lasting for 15 seconds, whether the mother feels the movement or not. Heart rate accelerations should be within 20 minutes of each other and within 40 minutes after monitoring begins. This is considered a **reactive nonstress test** and it is reassuring as to the status of the fetus. Tests can be **nonreactive**, normally up to 32 weeks gestation. A nonreactive test should prompt a re-test or possibly a contraction stress test or biophysical profile to determine fetal status.

Normal Fetal Breathing Movements Seen During Biophysical Profile

Researchers find that fetuses **breathe** in a discontinuous way, exhibiting paradoxical chest wall movement. Fetal breathing is required for proper lung development. Sighs or gasps are seen 1 to 4 times a minute. Irregular bursts of breaths also occur that have a rate of up to 240 cycles per minute. The fetal respiratory rate decreases between 33 and 36 weeks of gestation when the fetal lungs are finally mature.

Fetal breathing patterns in the final ten weeks of pregnancy vary according to time of day. Observations of fetal breathing activity must take this into consideration. Fetal breath rates increase after the mother eats a meal. It decreases in general in the evening from 7 pm to midnight, then increases to a peak from 4 am to 7 pm with a gradual decrease during the day.

Contraction Stress Test

A contraction stress test is one in which the reactivity of the FHR is compared with uterine contractions. Since contractions decrease blood flow to the fetus, additional stress from oligohydramnios, cord compression, or placental insufficiency will elicit late or variable FHR decelerations. If not already present, contractions are stimulated with 2 minutes of nipple stimulation by the mother or by an infusion of oxytocin. The goal is to observe 3 contractions within a 10-minute period to see how the fetal heart responds. A negative result is one in which no late or significant variable decelerations of the FHR occur. A suspicious test shows intermittent late decelerations or significant variable decelerations. A positive test shows late decelerations after half of the contractions.

Triple Test

The triple test is a screening tool that tests maternal blood for fetal chromosomal defects between gestational weeks 15 to 20. The test screens:

- **Alpha-fetoprotein (AFP)**: This protein is produced by the fetus.
- **Human chorionic gonadotropin (hCG)**: This hormone is produced by the placenta.
- **Unconjugated estriol (UE3)**: This estrogen is produced by the fetus and the placenta.

The results from the 3 tests are assessed together:

- **Trisomy 21 (Down syndrome)**: hcG is elevated and AFP and UE3 are low.
- **Trisomy 18 (Edwards' syndrome)**: levels of all 3 markers are low.
- **Neural tube defects/anencephaly**: AFP is elevated. (It's important that gestational age is correct for accuracy of test results.)

If abnormal findings occur, then further testing is indicated to confirm a diagnosis. These tests can include repeat blood screening, amniocentesis, percutaneous umbilical blood sampling, and ultrasound. Patients with confirmed diagnosis should be referred for genetic counseling.

Doppler Velocimetry During Pregnancy

The Doppler is used to measure the flow of red blood cells in maternal and fetal blood vessels. **Doppler studies** of the umbilical artery are used to monitor fetuses with growth restriction. Signs of absent or reversed end-diastolic flow in the umbilical artery can be caused by fetal aneuploidy, a severe anomaly, or severe fetal compromise, and may require immediate delivery. The Doppler is also used to monitor for constriction of the ductus arteriosus in fetuses exposed to indomethacin or other nonsteroidal anti-inflammatory drugs (NSAIDs). Uterine blood flow can be evaluated by Doppler for changes related to pregnancy-induced hypertension and impending preeclampsia.

MRI to Evaluate Fetus

Fetal magnetic resonance imaging (MRI) has been found to be a safe and excellent way to view nearly every part of the fetal anatomy in detail. Fast acquisition sequencing has solved the problems with fetal movement. MRI allows more accurate estimation of the fetal weight. Brain anomalies show up readily on fetal MRI, making this the most common use. The test is expensive and requires skill to obtain and to interpret; however, the results are superior to other methods of fetal assessment when details of the particular anomaly suspected are desired prior to birth.

Acid Base Assessment

Acoustic Stimulation and Scalp Stimulation

Acoustic stimulation uses loud noise to startle the fetus. FHR monitoring is done during the test to record accelerations in response to the sound stimulus. An **acoustic stimulator** delivers sound between 100 and 105 dB to the surface of the maternal abdomen. The sound is delivered for up to 3 seconds and repeated up to 3 times. **Scalp stimulation** is performed by placing firm pressure on the fetal head during a vaginal examination. The response of the FHR is then monitored. These tests take less time than a conventional nonstress test. About half of those fetuses that do not respond to acoustic stimulation or scalp stimulation are found to be acidotic so a negative test should prompt fetal scalp blood testing or plans for an emergency delivery.

FBS to Determine Fetal Blood Gas Status

Fetal scalp blood can be obtained to check blood gases of the fetus during labor when membranes have already ruptured and there is access to the scalp. The most important parameters used are those of pH and base excess. These results can be affected by many factors, including length of time drawing the sample, exposure to air, improper handling or technique, drawing a sample during a contraction, maternal position, fever, or hypertension, and the presence of caput succedaneum. A pH below 7 and base excess below -7 combined with signs of distress on electronic fetal heart monitor tracings will prompt an emergency birth. Fetal blood sampling requires skill and because

- 34 -

of many false-positives, it is used infrequently. Scalp stimulation is used more often to determine FHR reactivity as a sign of fetal status.

Value of Obtaining Umbilical Cord Blood Gases

Cord blood gases give a picture of the acid base status in the newborn's tissues at the time of birth. After birth, a segment of the umbilical cord is clamped on each end and placed on the delivery table until newborn status is determined. An accurate **pH and blood gas analysis** can be performed on this cord blood for up to 60 minutes after birth. ACOG recommends obtaining arterial and venous cord blood samples after cesarean sections for fetal distress, abnormalities during FHR evaluation in labor, low Apgar scores, growth restriction, maternal hypothyroidism, maternal fever, or multiple fetuses. When done rapidly after birth, the blood gas results can guide the treatment of the compromised neonate.

Electronic Fetal Monitoring

Fetal Pulse Oximetry During Labor

Studies continue to be done in an effort to define the role of **fetal pulse oximetry** in intrapartum fetal evaluation. A pad-like sensor is used to determine fetal pulse oximetry by placing it against the fetal face after membranes are ruptured. Fetal oxygen saturation has been found to vary greatly during labor when measured via umbilical blood. Saturation can fall to below 30% for brief periods during normal labors that have a good outcome. Signs of danger include saturation levels that remain below 30% for 2 minutes or longer.

FHR Baseline Variability, Absent Variability, Minimal Variability, Moderate Variability, and Marked Variability

FHR baseline variability is the difference in time interval from one heartbeat to the next and is seen as a wavering on the monitor tracing. It is a normal finding in a healthy fetus. **Absent variability** means that there is no discernible change in the baseline amplitude range. **Minimal variability** shows up as changes in the baseline amplitude that are less than 5 beats per minute. **Moderate variability** is defined as changes in the baseline amplitude that are between 6 and 25 beats per minute. **Marked variability** is present when the changes in the baseline amplitude are over 25 beats per minute.

NICHD Category I, II and III Fetal Heart Rate Tracings

NICHD Category fetal heart tracings assess acid-base status at the time of observation only, as fetal status may change over time and the fetus's category may change:

- **I (Normal)**: Tracings indicate baseline FHR of 110 to 160 bpm with only moderate variability. There may be early decelerations but no late or variable decelerations. This category predicts normal acid-base status.
- **II (indeterminate)**: May include numerous findings inconsistent with category I or I. Variability may be minimal or marked. Variability without recurrent decelerations may be absent. Accelerations after fetal stimulation may be absent. Deceleration may be prolonged, variable, or recurrent late with only moderate variability. Data is insufficient to categorize as I or II or to assume abnormal acid-base status.
- **III (abnormal)**: There is no variability in FHR with recurrent late decelerations, recurrent variable decelerations, or bradycardia. A sinusoidal pattern may be noted. This category predicts abnormal acid-base status.

- 35 -

FHR Baseline, Fetal Bradycardia, and Fetal Tachycardia

It is important to know the definitions of various terms pertaining to FHR monitoring. The **FHR baseline** is determined by looking at a 10-minute strip, and determining the baseline heart rate that is present for at least 2 minutes, and which varies by no more than 25 beats per minute. The baseline does not include any periodic or episodic changes or any marked variability. This rate is normally 110 to 160 beats per minute. **Fetal bradycardia** is a baseline rate that is less than 110 beats per minute. **Fetal tachycardia** is a baseline rate that is more than 160 beats per minute.

External FHR Monitoring

This method may be used prior to the rupture of membranes and dilatation of the cervix because it is noninvasive; however, it is not as accurate as internal monitoring. A transducer is strapped to the abdomen to pick up the sounds of the fetal heart valves and blood ejection during systole. The resultant FHR is then displayed on the monitor. A gel is used to obtain proper conduction of sound from the fetal heart to the transducer. Leopold maneuvers determine fetal lie; the transducer is then applied over the back or chest of the fetus. A tocodynamometer is used to monitor uterine activity to allow correlation between fetal heart activity and uterine contractions. This method is problematic in the obese patient. It is also affected by maternal position and movement and fetal movement. Fetal heart tones may not be reliably obtained during a contraction.

Internal Fetal Heart Monitor

An internal fetal heart monitor may be used when the membranes are ruptured and the cervix is dilated to 2 or 3 cm. A spiral electrode is screwed into the fetal scalp. This allows the FHR to be more accurately distinguished from the maternal heart beat. If fetal death has occurred, the maternal heart beat will be detected by the electrode. A reference electrode is attached to the maternal thigh. An intrauterine pressure monitoring catheter is inserted into the uterus next to the fetus to monitor contractions, allowing direct correlation between fetal heart activity and uterine contractions. Internal monitoring is the most accurate method of monitoring contractions and the FHR.

Interpreting FHR Patterns During Monitoring

First determine the **scale** used on the monitor. It affects the appearance of the FHR tracing and can distort patterns, resulting in erroneous **interpretation**. The recommended scaling to use is one that utilizes a vertical scale of 30 beats per minute with a range of 30 to 240 beats per minute. The recommended paper speed of 3 cm per minute results in a baseline that is smoother, making changes easier to see. Next, assess the 5 components of the **FHR monitor strip**: the baseline rate, any accelerations or decelerations of the FHR, any variability, any periodic or episodic changes in the baseline rate, and changes in the FHR pattern over time. Note any **unusual patterns** in the FHR. Report a sinusoidal heart rate, fetal arrhythmias, or marked variability to the physician or midwife. Determine the correlation of the FHR to contractions and report absence of accelerations or presence of decelerations.

Sinusoidal FHR Pattern

A sinusoidal FHR pattern is rare. It appears as a wavy line that oscillates evenly above and below the heart rate baseline in a regular fashion. The baseline is usually in the range of 110 to 160 beats per minute. The oscillations are from 5 to 15 beats per minute and occur at a frequency of 2 to 5 cycles per minute. Variability and reactivity is absent and there is no correlation of heart beat to contractions, fetal movement, or stimulation. This pattern accompanies severe fetal anemia caused

- 36 -

by Rh isoimmunization, placental abruption, or maternal-fetal hemorrhage. It is also caused by fetal cardiac anomalies, infection, and asphyxia. It signifies severe fetal distress and impending death. It may be reversed by a fetal transfusion in some cases. Assess the pattern for signs of variability, accelerations, and regularity of oscillations. Maternal butorphanol injection or fentanyl administration can cause a pseudo sinusoidal pattern, which includes variability, accelerations, and irregular oscillations. This is resolved with drug excretion.

FHR Monitoring of Preterm Fetuses and Term Fetuses

Premature fetuses differ in their heart rate patterns during labor from term fetuses. **FHR patterns** that are not reassuring are especially significant and signify fetal depression, hypoxemia, or acidemia in 70% to 80% of preterm infants before 33 weeks gestation versus 20% at term. Deterioration of the FHR occurs more often and more quickly in the premature infant; nonreassuring changes need to be identified and rapid action taken to intervene. Because premature fetuses that are born in a depressed state have a higher rate of morbidity and mortality, perinatal intervention is of critical importance. The baseline rate of the preterm fetus decreases as gestation increases. Variability is minimal to absent more often and predicts hypoxemia. Accelerations are lower in beats per minute and occur less frequently. Variable decelerations are more common during labor in the preterm fetus and are associated with hypoxemia.

Signs of Fetal Hypoxemia or Acidemia in FHR Tracing During Second-Stage Labor

Nearly all FHR tracings show "normal" decelerations during the second stage of labor from cord or head compression. Unfortunately, the unpredictability of FHR changes during the second stage of labor requires erring on the side of caution if prolonged changes in heart rate are seen prior to birth. The length of time that the fetus has a decelerated heart beat can be correlated to Apgar scores at 5 minutes. Frequent or long-term decelerations, baseline bradycardia or tachycardia, or loss of beat-to-beat variability often accompany **fetal acidemia**. The presence of these abnormalities on the FHR can signify fetal distress and the birth of a neonate who may require resuscitation upon delivery.

Monitoring of Multiple FHRs

Different fetuses rarely have matching FHRs, so differences should be distinguishable on the FHR tracings. Assess these tracings to determine that they are not from a single fetus. Fetuses may interact in the womb and cause simultaneous accelerations of heart rate. The mother can notify the nurse of movement that can then verify this kind of tracing. During labor, one fetus may be stable while another shows signs of distress via heart rate changes. Multiple gestations frequently result in a cesarean birth. Therefore, there is not much research concerning the changes in FHR in multiple fetuses during labor.

Artifacts on the Fetal Heart Rate Tracing

Various artifacts (misleading fetal heart tracings) can occur when monitoring fetal heart rate, usually related to the maternal heart rate, which results in **signal ambiguity** (maternal heart rate displayed on FHR monitor). Artifacts can result from:

- **Maternal pacemaker interference**: Fetal electrode may record pacemaker firing.
- **Deceased fetus**: The maternal heartbeat may continue to register on the fetal electrode.
- **Superimposition**: The maternal heart rate or QRS complex may be superimposed on the fetal heart tracing.
- **Maternal heart rate tracing** displayed instead of fetal.

Artifacts and signal ambiguity should be suspected when the fetal heart rates continues at a low normal rate, at least 50% of contractions result in accelerations of FHR, and the FHR appears to decelerate to the maternal heart rate and does not return to baseline. If signal ambiguity is expected, the maternal pulse rate should be counted and traced and fetal and maternal tracings compared. To correct, the FHR should be assessed with ultrasound, the Doppler sensor relocated, or a scalp electrode placed.

Early and Late Decelerations in the FHR on the Monitor Tracing

When decelerations of the FHR occur, the onset, nadir, and recovery of the deceleration should be compared with the beginning, peak, and ending of the nearest contraction. **Early decelerations** occur gradually over more than 30 seconds from onset to nadir. The onset, nadir, and recovery of the deceleration usually match the beginning, peak, and ending of the contraction. **Late decelerations** also occur gradually over more than 30 seconds from onset to nadir. However, the onset, nadir, and recovery of the deceleration occur later than the beginning, peak, and ending of the contraction.

Variable, Prolonged, and Recurrent Decelerations in the FHR on the Monitor Tracing

Variable decelerations occur abruptly over less than 30 seconds from onset to nadir. They are a decrease of at least 15 beats per minute or more from the baseline and last longer than 15 seconds but less than 2 minutes from onset to recovery. They vary in timing from one contraction to the next. **Prolonged decelerations** are a decrease of at least 15 beats per minute or more from the baseline and last longer than 2 minutes but less than 10 minutes from onset to recovery. **Recurrent decelerations** occur with at least half of the contractions seen on a 20-minute monitoring strip.

Early Decelerations of the FHR

Early decelerations occur gradually over more than 30 seconds from onset to nadir. The onset, nadir, and recovery of the deceleration usually match the beginning, peak, and ending of the contraction. They are thought to be caused by fetal head compression, which stimulates the fetal vagus nerve and results in a deceleration of the heart rate. To assess **early decelerations**, verify that they coincide with contractions and that normal variability in the FHR baseline is present. When these factors are present, the fetal status is considered stable without signs of hypoxia.

Late Decelerations of the FHR

Late decelerations occur gradually over more than 30 seconds from onset to nadir. The onset, nadir, and recovery of the deceleration occur later then the beginning, peak, and ending of the nearest contraction. They can occur during rapid descent, periods of maternal hypotension, or when the presenting head is in the occiput posterior position. They also occur when there is placental insufficiency with decreased fetal tolerance for the stress of labor, and are then considered a sign of hypoxia. Assess the amount of variability present in the baseline, since absent or minimal variability is ominous. **Late decelerations** may develop after a period of variable decelerations or other baseline rate changes.

Prolonged Decelerations of the FHR

Prolonged decelerations are an abrupt decrease of the FHR of at least 15 beats per minute or more from the baseline and last longer than 2 minutes but less than 10 minutes from onset to recovery. They usually occur as an isolated incident. They are thought to be caused by serious maternal respiratory, cardiac, or neurological distress, but are more commonly caused by cord compression,

- 38 -

uterine hyperstimulation, uterine or vasa previa rupture, or maternal hypotension. Vagal stimulation by pressure on the fetal skull can cause **prolonged decelerations** when the fetus is occiput posterior or in a transverse lie. Induction of regional anesthesia or a supine maternal position can also cause them. Assess the baseline and amount of variability before and after the incident to help determine whether the fetus is in distress. Normal baselines and variability are reassuring.

Accelerations and Prolonged Accelerations in the FHR on the Monitor Tracing

Acceleration in the FHR is observed as an abrupt rise from the baseline on a monitoring strip. Accelerations rise at least 15 beats per minute above the baseline heart rate, rise in less than 30 seconds to a peak rate, and last more than 15 seconds but less than 2 minutes from initial rise to the return to baseline. **Prolonged accelerations** rise at least 15 beats per minute above the baseline heart rate, rise in less than 30 seconds to a peak rate, and last more than 2 minutes but less than 10 minutes from initial rise to the return to baseline.

Absent or Minimal Variability of the FHR Baseline

Moderate variability is a reassuring sign of fetal well-being. Both undetectable variability and minimal variability (less than 5 beats per minute) cause concern. They can be caused by maternal drugs such as magnesium sulfate, analgesics, narcotics, or tranquilizers. Fetal acidemia can cause decreased variability and decelerations. Minimal variability may be seen during fetal sleep or when the fetus is premature. Cardiac or neurologic abnormalities also cause minimal variability. **Absent or minimal variability** should be evaluated without delay. An attempt to stimulate the fetus is made to see if the condition is temporary.

Significance of Marked Variability in the FHR Baseline

Marked FHR baseline variability that is over 25 beats per minute was known in the past as a salutatory pattern. It is thought to be the fetal response to sudden, brief episodes of hypoxia. It is uncommon and may be caused by uterine hyperstimulation or maternal ephedrine ingestion of 30 mg or more. Assess for the presence of decelerations. Marked variability is usually a response to hypoxia when abnormal FHR changes are also present. Changes in maternal position, administration of oxygen, and discontinuation of oxytocin are interventions for marked variability.

Variable Decelerations of the FHR

Variable decelerations occur abruptly over less than 30 seconds from onset to nadir. They are a decrease of at least 15 beats per minute or more from the baseline and last longer than 15 seconds but less than 2 minutes from onset to recovery. They vary in timing from one contraction to the next and can also accompany fetal movement. They are commonly seen during labor and are thought to be the result of cord compression; they happen more frequently when oligohydramnios is present. During the second stage of labor, they can be caused by the intense pressure on the fetal head and a rapid descent. A change in maternal position may alleviate the cord compression when variable decelerations are persistent. If it doesn't, more thoroughly assess the maternal-fetal status.

Assessment of Uterine Contractions

Uterine contraction assessment is correlated with the FHR to determine if labor is progressing normally. Contractions can be palpated with the hands. They can also be externally monitored by using a tocodynamometer or internally monitored by inserting an intrauterine pressure catheter after the membranes are ruptured and the cervix is dilated to 2 or 3 cm. Contractions should be

assessed for frequency (amount of time from the beginning of one contraction to the beginning of the next), duration (amount of time in seconds from the beginning to the end of the contraction), and intensity (mild, medium, or strong in strength). **Uterine resting tone** between contractions should also be determined. All four characteristics can be determined by palpation but it is a somewhat subjective method. External monitoring can determine the duration and frequency but not the intensity or resting tone. Internal monitoring is most accurate because the amniotic pressure is measured. It can be used to determine all four characteristics.

Abnormal Patterns of Uterine Activity

The desirable pattern of uterine activity during active labor is the presence of contractions every 2 to 3 minutes. Inadequate or abnormal patterns may develop, especially during oxytocin augmentation. A pattern of **hyperstimulation** is the persistence of more than 5 contractions in a 10-minute period or contractions that occur within 1 minute of each other. They may be caused by maternal hormones or agents used to ripen the cervix or augment labor. They can cause fetal distress by interfering with uteroplacental blood flow. **Coupling or tripling** occurs when contractions occur in groups of 2 or 3 with very little interval between, followed by a 2- to 5-minute rest period. This may occur as a result of incoordination of the uterine pacemakers or a decrease in sensitivity of oxytocin receptor sites in the uterine muscle.

Uterine Hypertonus and Uterine Tachysystole

Uterine hypertonus, a state in which the uterine muscle does not relax between contractions, may result from hormonal imbalance, immature genitals, infections, cervical failure, and fibroid tumors. Ineffectual contractions in the latent phase of labor become more frequent but do not result in dilation or effacement. The resting tone of the myometrium increases. The contractions may interfere with uteroplacental exchange, resulting in fetal distress. The pressure on the fetal head may result in cephalhematoma, caput succedaneum, or excessive molding. Oxytocin infusion or amniotomy may be used for treatment after assessment for cephalo-pelvic disproportion (CPD). **Uterine tachysystole** is 6 or more contractions in a 10-minute period (averaged over 30 minutes) or a series of 2-minute or greater single contractions. Common causes include infection, dehydration, placental abruption, and induction. While associated with fetal heart decelerations, the fetus does not generally suffer adverse effects unless the uterine tachysystole is associated with hypertonus.

Arrhythmias of the FHR

The FHR sometimes includes skips during pregnancy. These skips represent **extrasystoles** and usually resolve before or shortly after birth. They usually do not cause further problems. Evaluate the neonate after birth and perform a cardiac workup if a **tachyarrhythmia** persists. When arrhythmias persist during pregnancy, a fetal echocardiograph is done to evaluate the fetal heart. Supraventricular tachycardia may reach rates of 240 beats per minute. Heart block can cause **bradyarrhythmias** in the fetus. Careful maternal administration of antiarrhythmic drugs may be attempted. Assess the tracing for signs of artifact that confuses signs of fetal cardiac arrhythmia.

Fetal Tachycardia

Fetal tachycardia occurs when the FHR baseline rises above 160 beats per minute for at least 10 minutes. Assess the amount of variability and whether there are any decelerations before interpreting **fetal tachycardia**. Fetal acidemia is not usually present if there is at least moderate variability and no decelerations. Notify the physician of the need for evaluation if there is absent variability, or decelerations that are variable or late. Fetal tachycardia is often due to maternal

- 40 -

infection, fever, dehydration, or hyperthyroidism. Fetal causes include prematurity, infection, anemia, hypoxia, supraventricular tachycardia, or cardiac anomalies. Maternal medication with terbutaline or ritodrine causes both maternal and fetal tachycardia.

Fetal Bradycardia

Fetal bradycardia occurs when the FHR baseline falls below 110 beats per minute for at least 10 minutes. Assess the presence or absence of variability. A sudden, dramatic drop in the FHR occurs in the presence of fetal hypoxemia, rupture of a vasa previa, placental abruption, or a prolapsed umbilical cord. It is also a warning of uterine rupture if a woman is in labor following a previous cesarean birth. Maternal death can follow quickly unless delivery occurs without delay. **Fetal bradycardia** is not as well tolerated by the fetus if it was preceded by severe variable and late decelerations.

Injuries That Can Result from Electronic Fetal Monitoring

Occasionally, a fetal scalp electrode can cause **injury** to the fetal face during application if the presenting part is not accurately identified. It can also cause lacerations of the scalp. A placental blood vessel may be injured during insertion of an intrauterine catheter or the placenta or uterine wall may be punctured. The catheter may become entangled with the fetus, causing injury. Internal monitoring can result in infection of both mother and fetus. Therefore, ACOG advises that internal monitoring not be used if maternal HIV, herpes simplex virus, or hepatitis B or C virus is present.

Intermittent Auscultation During Labor

A **Doppler** may be used to monitor the FHR at **intervals** instead of continuously during labor in low-risk patients. This method of FHR monitoring should not be used during induction or augmentation of labor. The patient will need to be given 1:1 care to allow the nurse to monitor heart tones at a moment's notice as needed. FHR should be assessed every 30 minutes during the first stage, every 15 minutes during the second stage, and as needed. When risk factors are present, they should be assessed every 15 minutes in the first stage and every 5 minutes in the second stage, or continuous electronic fetal monitoring should be used.

Labor and Delivery

Labor Initiation

Maternal and Uteroplacental Physiological Changes During Labor

A number of maternal and uteroplacental physiological changes occur during labor. At the **onset of labor** (term), progesterone (which inhibits contractions) levels fall and estrogen levels increase, allowing the uterus to contract in response to the pituitary gland's release of oxytocin. The contractions put pressure on the cervix, resulting in dilation and effacement. At term, about 10% of cardiac output feeds the uterus, but uterine blood flow decreases during contractions (50% with 30 mm Hg pressure). If the amniotic sac did not rupture before onset of labor, it usually does so when dilation is complete. **After delivery** of the neonate, the uterus continues to contract, reducing bleeding and resulting in separation of the placenta from the uterine wall. The placenta is usually delivered within 30 minutes of birth. Post-partum uterine contractions continue for several hours, limiting blood loss, and facilitating involution (decreases from 1000 g weight at term to 100 g by week 3) and allowing other organs to return to their pre-pregnant positions.

Factors That May Initiate Labor

Fetal

The initiation of uterine contractions depends on both maternal and fetal factors. Fetal factors include:

- The **prostaglandin levels** rise when the amnion, chorion, and decidua release stored arachidonic acid that is converted to prostaglandin. The oxytocin receptors in the decidua prompt the continual release of arachidonic acid throughout labor, keeping prostaglandin levels high.
- The **placenta** ages and this triggers contractions.
- The release of **fetal cortisol** from the fetal adrenal glands reduces progesterone formation by the placenta and raises prostaglandin levels.
- The fetus secretes **oxytocin** equal to an infusion at 3 milliunits/min that helps to sustain labor.

Maternal

The initiation of uterine contractions depends on both maternal and fetal factors.

Maternal factors include:

- **Stretching of uterine muscles** causes a release of prostaglandin. Prostaglandin prepares the uterine muscle tissue to respond to oxytocin.
- **Decreased progesterone levels** allow estrogen to excite the uterine muscle response.
- **Cervical pressure** stimulates nerve plexus, resulting in signals to the posterior pituitary gland to release oxytocin.
- **Oxytocin release** into the circulation raises dramatically all throughout labor, peaking during the second stage. Along with prostaglandin, oxytocin keeps muscles from binding calcium. This raises the level of calcium in the blood, causing contractions to begin. Myometrial and decidual oxytocin receptors in the uterus increase in number towards the end of pregnancy. Myometrial receptors are thought to be important to the initiation of labor.

- 42 -

True Labor

When true labor begins, contractions may start out irregular than become regular within a short period of time. The strength and frequency increase and the intervals between contractions shorten until contractions are 2 to 3 minutes apart. Bloody show may occur and cervical dilatation occurs over time. The mother feels back pain that extends around to the abdomen. Walking and activity increases contractions and they do not stop during sleep. Maternal sedation does not stop contractions from occurring. Cervical effacement and dilatation occur gradually and steadily until the fetus is able to descend into the pelvis and birth occurs.

False Labor

During false labor, the contractions start out regular but decrease in strength and frequency, gradually lengthening the intervals between contractions. The mother feels discomfort in her groin and the lower part of the uterus. There is not usually a bloody show and no changes occur to the cervix. Contractions may decrease if the mother is active and stop during sleep. Contractions can be stopped via maternal sedation. Premonitory signs that may occur around this time include dropping of the fetus, pelvic pressure, frequency of urination, changes in vaginal discharges, loss of the cervical mucus plug, or a bloody show. Sleep changes and increased energy levels also occur.

Labor Management

Admission Assessment of Labor Patient

Most facilities use a form to help obtain the information for an **admission assessment**. A complete history and physical should be available from the physician or midwife, as well as progress notes from prenatal visits. Update the information since the last visit. This record should contain the previous obstetrical history, medical history, and history of this pregnancy. Symptoms of any current illnesses need to be noted. A thorough medical assessment is needed if there has been no prenatal care. Maternal vital signs, FHR, and the presence of uterine contractions as well as their frequency, intensity, and duration are noted. A vaginal exam is done to reveal whether any dilatation or effacement has occurred and whether membranes have ruptured. The presenting part and station are also determined. The physician or midwife is notified immediately if a fever, vaginal bleeding, acute abdominal pain, premature rupture of membranes, hypertension, or FHR changes are present. Urine is checked for protein and glucose.

Assessments of Mother and Fetus During Labor

Assessments of the mother and fetus during labor include taking the mother's vital signs, assessing uterine contraction strength, duration, and frequency, and assessing changes in the FHR as correlated with uterine contractions. The mother's pain and discomfort and response to labor are assessed. A vaginal exam is done as needed to determine dilatation, effacement, and station. Intake and output is measured and recorded. The rate of oxytocin or magnesium sulfate is verified and changed if warranted, and the response and any side effects are noted. During active labor these assessments are done every 30 minutes to 1 hour. When oxytocin or magnesium sulfate is used, assessments are done every 15 minutes and whenever the rate is changed with summaries every 30 minutes. When cervical ripening agents are used, assess every 30 minutes for 2 hours then every hour. Assessments are done every 15 minutes during the active pushing phase of the second stage of labor.

Vaginal Examination Procedure

Explain the procedure to the woman. Cleanse the perineum with warm water prior to the exam. Do not use povidone-iodine, hexachlorophene, or other antiseptics to cleanse. Use water-soluble lubricants and sterile gloves on thoroughly washed hands. Position the woman on her back with the head of the bed up slightly and expose the area only as necessary. Assess **dilatation and effacement** first. The cervix is normally 3.5 to 4 cm long prior to effacement. Find the ischial spines at the 3 or 9 o'clock position and 1 in deep in the vaginal walls, and then determine the station of the fetal head in relationship. **Engagement** of the fetal head (zero station) occurs when the occiput of the fetal head is at the level of the spines. Be sure to assess the level of the bony skull and not the caput formation. Finish by identifying the suture lines and fontanels to determine the fetal head position.

Assessments of Mother and Baby Immediately Postpartum

Assess the **vital signs** of the mother every 15 minutes for 1 hour or more frequently if complications occur. Assess uterine firmness and vaginal bleeding frequently and massage as needed. **Apgar scores** are obtained at 1 and 5 minutes after birth. They may be obtained every 5 minutes thereafter if the initial scores are less than 7. After initial care is given at birth, the newborn is assessed every 30 minutes until vital signs have been stable for at least 2 hours. The newborn's vital signs, color, peripheral circulation, respiratory efforts, level of consciousness, activity, and tone are all noted with intervention taken as needed.

Leopold Maneuvers

The four Leopold maneuvers are as follows:

- **First maneuver**: The presentation is determined by palpating the uterine fundus. A large nodular mass is the infant's buttocks, whereas a hard, round, ballottable, mobile mass is the fetal head.
- **Second maneuver**: Deep palpation of both sides of the maternal abdomen will determine where the fetal back is and whether it is oriented anteriorly, transversely, or posteriorly.
- **Third maneuver**: Using the thumb and fingers, the lower portion of the abdomen is grasped just above the symphysis pubis. The presenting part is palpated to see if it is moveable or engaged deeply into the pelvis.
- **Fourth maneuver**: The tips of the fingers are used to palpate deeply into the pelvic inlet to determine details of engagement.

Four Stages of Labor

The **first stage of labor** is divided into three phases. The first is the *latent phase*, during which the nulliparous woman completely effaces and dilatation to 3 cm occurs. (Effacement and dilatation occur simultaneously in multiparous women.) The second phase is the *active phase*, during which dilatation progresses to 7 cm. *Transition* is the phase during which dilatation to 10 cm is completed. The **second stage of labor** then begins. The *initial latent phase* of the second stage encompasses passive fetal descent and laboring down. The *active pushing phase* then occurs. The **third stage of labor** begins after the birth of the baby and ends when the placenta is delivered. The **fourth stage of labor** begins after the delivery of the placenta and ends when the mother is finally stabilized about 1-2 hours after birth.

First Stage

Latent phase: This **first phase of the first stage** lasts about 8.6 hours for primigravida and about 5.3 hours for multigravida. The cervix begins to dilate and efface in the multigravida at the same time. In the primigravida, the cervix dilates and effacement occurs before the second stage begins. The cervix in both women dilates to 3 cm. Contractions may be irregular, lasting 30 to 40 seconds, from 3 to 30 minutes apart, and of mild intensity by palpation and 25 to 40 mm Hg by intrauterine monitor. Bloody show may occur, membranes may rupture, and the woman may have diarrhea. Abdominal cramps of menstrual-like intensity and a low, moderate backache accompany the contractions. During this phase the mother controls the pain and is able to be active. She may feel excited and confident or anxious and worried about her upcoming labor and delivery.

Active phase: This **second phase of the first stage** lasts about 4.6 hours for primigravidas and about 2.4 hours for multigravida. The cervix dilates to 7 cm. Contractions are regular, lasting 40 to 60 seconds, from 2 to 5 minutes apart, and of moderate intensity by palpation and 50 to 70 mm Hg by intrauterine monitor. The contractions increase in discomfort along with pressure on the bladder and rectum. The woman's legs may tremble. When the fetus is in the occipitoposterior position, there is a persistent backache. The woman now concentrates on getting through contractions and is willing to work with the suggestions of those around her. She is less talkative during this stage as she conserves her strength.

Transition phase: This **third phase of the first stage** lasts about 3.6 hours for primigravidas and varies for multigravida. The cervix dilates to 10 cm and effacement is complete. Contractions are regular, lasting 60 to 90 seconds, from 1.5 to 2 minutes apart, and of strong intensity by palpation and 70 to 90 mm Hg by intrauterine monitor. There is an increase in rectal pressure and the woman feels the urge to push. Bloody show increases and the membranes may rupture if they have remained intact until now. The woman intensely concentrates on contractions and pushing, and she sleeps or rests between contractions. She may be fatigued, irritable, discouraged, and in need of support to help her get through this phase.

Second Stage

This second stage of labor lasts about 3 hours for primigravidas and up to 30 minutes for multigravida. The cervix is dilated, effacement is complete, and passive descent of the fetus occurs first in the initial latent phase. Then the active pushing phase continues until birth occurs. Contractions are regular, lasting 40 to 60 seconds, from 2 to 3 minutes apart, and of strong intensity by palpation and 70 to 100 mm Hg by intrauterine monitor. The woman feels an increasing rectal and perineal pressure and urge to push. The perineum burns and vaginal and perineal stretching occurs with tearing possible. The woman is intent on pushing and requires information and encouragement through the entire stage. She is eager to see the baby and know that all is well.

Third and Fourth Stages

The third stage of labor lasts from 5 to 30 minutes. It is the period of time from the birth of the baby to the birth of the placenta. The woman feels mild uterine contractions and fullness in the birth canal as the placenta is expelled from the uterus and vagina. She is concentrated upon the infant and her pride and relief in the completed birth.

The **fourth stage** begins after the birth of the placenta and lasts until the woman is stabilized, usually one to two hours after the birth. She may be anxious about tears and injury to her vagina and perineum. There may be pain as the perineum is anesthetized for repairs and repairs are completed. Recovery room care is given and the woman feels pain from uterine cramping and perineal repairs. She may have the urge to void and wish to eat and drink. She explores the infant

- 45 -

and interacts with her family to celebrate the birth. She may wish to nurse and experiences the letdown reflex.

Factors Contributing to Length of First Stage of Labor

The length of labor is affected by the use of methods to ripen the cervix and stimulate contractions. It is affected by the use of analgesics and anesthetics as well. The mother's weight and weight of the fetus affect labor. Smoking is less common among pregnant women. All of these factors combine to cause a **longer average length of labor** than that of the past. Parity affects the length of labor as do dosages of analgesia or anesthesia, rupture of membranes, labor and delivery positions, maternal pelvic anatomy, age, and psyche. The position and size of the fetus are also determinant factors in labor length. In general, nulliparous women dilate at a rate of 0.5 to 1 cm per hour and multiparous women dilate at a rate of more than 1 cm per hour.

Factors Contributing to Length of Second Stage of Labor

It used to be thought that the second stage of labor should be limited to 2 hours or less. The ability to use electronic fetal monitoring and epidural anesthetic has changed this timeline. It is permissible to allow the fetus to descend **at its own speed** providing that there are no changes in the FHR that signify distress and descent continues to occur. ACOG recommends that an operative vaginal birth be considered for nulliparous women with or without regional anesthesia if there are no signs of fetal descent for 2 hours. It should be considered for multiparas if there is no descent for 2 hours with regional anesthesia or for 1 hour without. Each mother-baby pair is unique and a thorough assessment of all factors involved helps guide the management of the second stage of labor for each pair.

Use of Fundal Pressure During Second Stage of Labor

There are few instances when fundal pressure during the second stage of labor may be used. It may be helpful during fetal scalp electrode application if the fetal station makes this difficult. It may be used to push the fetal head into the pelvis and against the cervix if membranes rupture before engagement occurs and there is a risk of a prolapsed cord. During birth, **fundal pressure** can be used when the head is crowning, FHR is nonreassuring, and the maternal effort is insufficient for birth to occur. The nurse has the right to refuse to participate in applying fundal pressure for the purpose of shortening the second stage without cause or during shoulder dystocia. Inappropriate fundal pressure can cause severe fetal complications such as shoulder impaction, brachial plexus injury, spinal cord injury, subgaleal hemorrhage when vacuum extraction is used, hypoxemia, and asphyxia. Maternal complications from fundal pressure include perineal lacerations and sphincter tears, uterine rupture and uterine inversion, pain, bruising, rib fracture, liver damage, hypotension, and respiratory distress.

Proper Method of Pushing

The individual woman's urge to **push** should be honored rather than making her wait until she is fully dilated. Her urge is due to the **Ferguson reflex** that occurs when the presenting fetal part begins to stretch the muscles of the pelvic floor. Restrain from teaching the typical closed-glottis method for 10 seconds since this uses the Valsalva maneuver that is adverse for both mother and fetus. Teach the woman to keep her feet flat on the bed while pushing and to not force her legs against her abdomen to avoid perineal nerve damage. Coach the woman to bear down for as long as she feels she can when she feels the urge to push and to take several breaths between bearing-down efforts. Women will normally use both closed- and open-glottis pushing during the second stage. Gentle, natural pushing is easier on the fetus and more appropriate. Urge her to continue to push for as long as she feels is comfortable and only when she has the urge.

Providing Emotional Support During Labor and Delivery

The laboring mother depends on the nurse to provide information so that she will know what to expect, how to interpret physical sensations, and how to lessen pain, breathe, and relax during her labor and delivery. She also needs to know that the nurse is monitoring her fetus' well-being. Nursing support that is caring, individual, and competent results in a more satisfying birth experience for the mother. Allowing the woman to choose the family members or other support persons who will be with her during labor and delivery is important to family-centered care during this time. Constant **support** lessens pain, maternal and fetal complications, and dissatisfaction with the birthing experience. It can also enhance family bonding to the newborn and provides a birthing experience that is unique to that family.

Provision of Food and Fluids During Labor and Birth

Fasting during labor was thought to be necessary to prevent aspiration pneumonitis in the case of a cesarean section. It is now known that even when fasting there will be acid contents in the stomach and fasting only increases the concentration. Decreased use of general anesthesia, cricoid pressure, improved intubation techniques, and administration of antacids has decreased the incidences of aspiration. Therefore, unless there are risks of complications, the laboring woman may usually **eat or drink**. The mother needs **50 to 100 calories per hour of labor** taken in small amounts of food. Clear fluids are allowed. IV Ringer's lactate may be given instead of food or fluids, or in the case of fetal distress to increase placental perfusion. IV glucose solutions are avoided since they can cause fetal hyperglycemia, reactive hypoglycemia, and other problems in the neonate. Studies suggest that the woman needs 250 mL/h of IV fluids during labor to prevent complications of labor caused by dehydration.

Principles of Active Management of Labor

Active management of labor refers to the shortening of labor via amniotomy and oxytocin augmentation. It is a controversial protocol developed in Ireland and evaluated in the United States. It requires 1:1 care by a labor nurse. It is used for nulliparous women in spontaneous, active labor. The pregnancy must be a single one, with a cephalic presentation, and with no signs of fetal distress present. Contractions must be active with bloody show, rupture of membranes, or 100% cervical effacement present to represent true labor. An amniotomy is done if membranes do not rupture within 1 hour after true labor is recognized. An oxytocin infusion is begun if dilatation is not progressing at 1 cm per hour. The rate is increased every 15 minutes until adequate contractions occur, to a maximum dose of 40 milliunits/min. There is a risk of uterine hyperstimulation and fetal distress from this technique.

Importance of Maternal Positioning During Labor and Birth

The woman's culture, physician's preference, and birthing unit norms all impact **positions during labor and delivery**. Women may be confined to bed because of monitoring requirements but can change positions in bed. Ambulation and mobility increases the woman's comfort, tolerance of labor, and can shorten labor. Electronic fetal monitoring (EFM) via telemetry allows both mobility and monitoring capabilities. An upright position of 30 degrees is helpful during labor and delivery. Squatting decreases the length of the second stage along with the number of lacerations, episiotomies, and operative vaginal births, compared with recumbent births. The supine position is avoided to prevent maternal hypotension from the pressure of the uterus. A left or right side lying

- 47 -

position may be taken for comfort. A hands-and-knees position may help the fetus to turn, relieve back pain during labor, or be used during delivery. Birthing balls may be used to help the woman find a comfortable position. A towel may also be used during pushing, with a nurse holding one end and the mother holding the other.

Enhancing Maternal and Family Bonding

When neonatal conditions allow, **skin-to-skin contact** between mother and baby directly after birth increases and helps to regulate neonatal temperature, and helps prevent hypoglycemia. The breastfeeding experience is enhanced by allowing the neonate to smell the mother's skin and breast milk odor as soon as possible after birth and by encouraging breastfeeding as early as possible. It encourages the mother's sense of responsibility towards the newborn. Allowing the mother to have those she desires with her for the labor and delivery of her baby helps to individualize the birth experience and make it satisfying to her and her family. The ability to see and touch the newborn soon after birth allows family members to **bond** with the baby. Siblings who are properly prepared can benefit from labor and birth attendance if it is integrated as a positive caretaking experience.

Professional Doula

A doula can fill the laboring mother's need for constant support when the labor nurse and father are not enough. **Doulas** are professionally trained to be support persons during pregnancy, labor, birth, and postpartum period. They enhance the woman's feeling of safety and confidence in her care during labor and delivery. The help of a doula can result in a shorter labor, decreased need for pain medication, augmentation, and operative births, and a positive neonatal outcome. She can visit the new family in the home setting and be a resource during this period. She helps the woman integrate the birth experience more fully by providing missing details, praising her efforts during labor and birth, and helping her understand any untoward events that occurred. There is less anxiety and distress in the mother and family and more pride and satisfaction in the entire birthing experience.

Obstetrical Procedures

Methods Used to Cause Cervical Ripening

Pharmacological

Pharmacological methods for **cervical ripening** include the application of prostaglandin E_1 (PGE_1), misoprostol (Cytotec), or dinoprostone (PGE_2) preparations to the cervix. Dinoprostone (PGE_2) is approved by the FDA for cervical ripening. Misoprostol is not yet approved by the FDA for this use. However, its low cost, efficacy, and ease of insertion encourage its use. Prostaglandin preparations soften the cervix, relax cervical smooth muscle, and induce contractions. The uterus then responds more readily to oxytocin inducement with coordinated contractions. Since prostaglandins promote uterine activity, they are considered the first step in labor induction.

Mechanical

Mechanical methods of **cervical ripening** include the insertion of Laminaria, synthetic dilators, or balloon catheters into the cervix to widen it gradually, promoting the initiation of contractions. Mechanical methods cause a lower risk of uterine hyperstimulation than pharmacological methods. They are used during a trial of labor for vaginal birth after prior cesarean (VBAC) for this reason. Mechanical dilators are inserted into the cervix when there is little or no cervical effacement. They are left in place for 6 to 12 hours and then removed. A vaginal exam is done to check the progress of ripening. If needed, fresh dilators can then be inserted if the cervix is not yet ripe.

- 48 -

Membrane Stripping and Amniotomy

Membrane stripping is performed by inserting one finger into the cervical opening and rotating it 360 degrees. This action separates the chorioamnionic membrane from the wall of the cervix and lower part of the uterus, releasing prostaglandins from the amnion, chorion, and decidua. It may also stimulate the posterior pituitary gland to secrete oxytocin. **Membrane stripping** works well for a nulliparous woman with an unripe cervix.

Uterine Hyperstimulation

Hyperstimulation is the persistence of more than 5 contractions in a 10-minute period or contractions that occur within 1 minute of each other. They may be caused by maternal hormones or agents used to ripen the cervix or augment labor, such as oxytocin. They can cause fetal distress by interfering with uteroplacental blood flow and oxygen supply to the fetus. Over time, fetal metabolic acidosis occurs and the FHR pattern changes to become nonreassuring. **Hyperstimulation** should be treated as soon as it occurs to prevent fetal distress. The mother is repositioned and a bolus of Ringer's lactate solution is given. Reduce oxytocin infusions to half the dosage and discontinue them if normal uterine contraction pattern has not recurred within 10 minutes. When hyperstimulation has resolved and the FHR is reassuring, the oxytocin infusion is restarted after stoppage for less than 30 minutes at half the rate that caused the hyperstimulation, or at the initial level if stopped for more than 30 minutes.

Administration of Oxytocin

Following the facility policy, **oxytocin** is piggy-backed into a main IV line nearest the patient. It is diluted according to policy to various strengths. Computations of drip rates must take the strength into consideration. The nurse must regulate the infusion rate according to the physician's orders and the response of the fetus and mother. The rate is increased if no response and decreased if contractions are too frequent or if there are nonreassuring changes in the FHR. Uterine hyperstimulation and dysfunctional uterine activity patterns can result from long-term infusion at higher than appropriate doses. When active labor is established, the infusion of oxytocin is stopped.

Bishop Score

The Bishop score uses the assessment of 5 parameters to determine readiness of the cervix for **induction** with higher scores being more favorable. Cervical dilatation is assessed and assigned a score of 0 for no dilatation, 1 for dilatation of 1 to 2 cm, 2 for dilatation of 3 to 4 cm, and 3 for dilatation of 5 cm or more. Cervical effacement is assessed and assigned a score of 0 for 0% to 30% effacement, 1 for 40% to 50%, 2 for 60% to 70%, and 3 for 80% or more. Fetal station is assigned a score of 0 for a -3 station, 1 for -2, 2 for -1 to 0, and 3 for +1 or +2 station. Cervical consistency is rated 0 for firm, 1 for moderate, and 2 for a soft consistency. Cervical position is rated 0 for posterior, 1 for midposition, and 2 for anterior. A Bishop score of 6 or more predicts the start of spontaneous labor within 7 days.

Augmentation of Labor

Augmentation is performed when labor progress is slower than normal (protracted) or contractions stop (arrest) after the active stage of labor has been reached. All factors must be considered, including analgesia given, size of the fetus and pelvis, and presentation. An oxytocin infusion is used at a lower rate than that used for induction of labor. If labor fails to reestablish at a normal rate, a cesarean birth may be considered. There is controversy regarding the use of high doses of oxytocin to augment labor. It is thought that less oxytocin should be needed for

- 49 -

augmentation since there is less resistance in the cervix. The response of each woman seems to be individualized, and depends on previous spontaneous uterine activity and sensitivity to oxytocin at the time of the augmentation efforts.

Induction of Woman Who Has Had a VBAC

Women who have had a **previous cesarean birth** (VBAC) may choose to undergo a trial of labor to see if normal dilatation and effacement occur without threatening the mother or fetus. It is best if labor onset is spontaneous. Induction using pharmacologic agents increases the risk of uterine rupture at the site of the old scar. This is higher with the use of prostaglandins; therefore, ACOG recommends the use of oxytocin alone. Maternal and fetal status is closely evaluated throughout the trial of labor. Uterine rupture results in massive hemorrhage that threatens the life of the mother and fetus immediately. A repeat cesarean is performed if there are any signs of distress in either party.

Version Procedures

Version alters the fetal presentation through manipulation. **External cephalic version** is recommended for breech presentation and transverse lie if the position is recognized prior to onset of labor, gestation is about 36 weeks (small fetus), and vaginal delivery is an option. Contraindications include placenta previa and non-reassuring fetal status. Prior Caesarean is a relative contraindication. Version is most successful if there is adequate amnionic fluid, unengaged fetus, and tocolysis. The nurse must monitor the fetal heart rate during the procedure. Version is stopped if the heart rate becomes abnormal. Procedure: For a forward roll, one hand is placed externally over the fetal head and one on the fetal buttocks. The buttocks are lifted in a clockwise direction toward the fundus while the head is guided toward the pelvis. If this is unsuccessful, then a backward flip can be attempted. The version is successful if the head remains above the symphysis pubis. Complications are rare but can include premature rupture of membranes, placentae abruptio, and obstruction of umbilical cord.

Perineal Lacerations

First degree: The perineal skin and the mucous membranes of the vagina are torn.

Second degree: The perineal skin and vaginal mucous membranes are torn as well as the fascia and muscle of the perineum.

Third degree: The perineal skin, vaginal mucous membranes, and fascia and muscle of the perineum are torn and the tear extends into the rectal sphincter.

Fourth degree: The perineal skin, vaginal mucous membranes, and fascia and muscle of the perineum are torn, the tear extends into the rectal sphincter, and the inner lumen of the rectum is exposed.

Episiotomies

The rate of episiotomy use has declined. It is thought that birth without **episiotomy** results in less blood loss, a lower infection rate, and reduced perineal pain in the postpartum period. The physician or midwife's beliefs and experience influence their use of episiotomies to prevent tearing, to improve the ease of perineal repair, to reduce stress on the fetal head, and to allow more room for a breech or operative vaginal birth. Techniques to avoid perineal tearing and the need for an episiotomy include upright position for pushing, gentle open-glottis pushing, pushing only when the urge is felt, allowing time for passive fetal descent and gradual stretching of the perineum, and birthing between contractions.

Perioperative Nursing Care for Cesarean Birth

Several professional organizations have standards, recommendations, and guidelines to be followed when writing the hospital policies and procedures that govern perio**perative care of the woman who has a cesarean birth**. They include the Joint Commission, the Association of Perioperative Registered Nurses (AORN), the American Society of Perianesthesia Nurses (ASPAN), the American Academy of Pediatrics (AAP), the American College of Obstetricians and Gynecologists (ACOG), the American Heart Association (AHA), and the American Society of Anesthesiologists (ASA). Standards dictate that any facility offering labor and delivery services must be ready to perform an emergency cesarean section within 30 minutes. If the cesarean is performed in a labor and delivery suite instead of a hospital operating suite, the same standards must be followed as though it were in the operating room (OR). Perioperative nursing care must also be the same. The same equipment is required as in the OR. Personnel must be available at the birth to care for both mother and baby and must be skilled in resuscitation.

Controversy About Cesarean Birth Without Medical Indication

Some physicians believe that women have the right to request a cesarean birth when there is no **medical indication**. The number of these requested cesareans has increased in number. They may not be covered by insurance reimbursement. Gestational age and lung maturity of the fetus must be determined prior to elective cesarean birth. There is a higher risk of postpartum hemorrhage and a longer hospital stay required. There is a slightly higher risk of infections, anesthesia complications, placenta previa, and impaired breastfeeding. Cesarean birth may avoid uterine rupture in those with a cesarean scar, and the number of bladder problems, pelvic organ prolapse, and anorectal problems are decreased slightly over vaginal birth. Neonates have increased respiratory problems with cesarean birth. There is slightly lower incidence of fetal intracranial hemorrhage, asphyxia, brain damage, birth injury, and infection in the neonate after cesarean birth. Evidence for and against requested cesarean birth must continue to be gathered before policy addresses this situation.

Intraoperative Care for Cesarean Birth

The woman is lying supine with a wedge under one hip. Fetal monitoring should continue until the abdomen is ready to be prepped for surgery and then the monitors are removed. A grounding device is employed. The woman's vital signs, FHR, abdominal skin status, and her emotional state are documented. Personnel and equipment for baby care are verified. Family members are assisted into position and directions are given. The nurse assists the anesthesiologist and mother as needed when anesthesia is administered. Circulating nurse duties are performed, including sponge, needle, and other equipment counts. The nurse applies a dressing to the wound, documents maternal and neonatal status, and transports the woman to the postanesthesia care unit (PACU).

Report from PACU Nurse to Postpartum Nurse Concerning Cesarean Birth

Areas that should be covered in the report from the **PACU nurse** to the **postpartum nurse** include the following: allergies, medications and fluids given including anesthesia and pain, I & O totals, blood loss, vital signs, level of care, neuromuscular status, operative incision type and dressing condition, fundal height and firmness, lochia, perineal condition if vaginal birth was attempted prior to the cesarean, locations of IVs, drainage tubes or catheters, pain assessments and interventions used, presence of nausea or vomiting, laboratory work, family and neonatal

- 51 -

information, status of breastfeeding attempts, any bonding that occurred, postpartum plans for rooming-in or adoption, publicity wishes of the patient, orders for postpartum care, and information about the maternal and neonatal physicians.

Supporting Maternal Bonding After Cesarean Birth

Women who have a cesarean, whether planned or emergent, need information throughout the process to help relieve anxiety. When possible, having the same nurse during the entire experience can help create trust. The mother needs to be given choices and control over care when possible to help make her experience more satisfying. Honoring her wish for sustained contact with the newborn helps her to accept the change in birth plans and experience. The presence of family or a support person during the cesarean and afterwards helps to make the experience more family-oriented and less stressful for the mother. The family can help the mother to safely care for the baby in her postpartum room even when she has had analgesia or needs to rest. This enhances bonding and breastfeeding.

Current Rate of Cesarean Births in US

The rate of cesarean births has risen to its highest ever in the United States. In the 1990s, the VBAC rate increased but it has since decreased because of various factors. Up to 90% of women who had one cesarean birth will have another during subsequent pregnancies. Medical complications, nonreassuring FHRs, and placenta previa are the most common medical indications. Lack of progress in labor or arrests of labor are also indications. Cesarean birth is more common when a nulliparous woman is induced prior to the start of spontaneous labor and inductions of this type are occurring more often these days. Some women request a cesarean birth without any medical indication and this raises the rates as well.

Postanesthesia Recovery Care for Cesarean Birth

Postanesthesia care is given according to PACU standards. The intraoperative course is reviewed with the circulating nurse. Maternal assessments in the PACU include vital signs, respiratory, circulation, neuromuscular, and obstetrical status, level of consciousness, I & O (intake and output), pain level, and interaction between the mother and baby if present, as well as the status of the neonate. All assessments are documented. PACU discharge criteria are followed to determine when she may be released to the postpartum care area. The anesthesiologist must sign her release from PACU. She is transferred to postpartum care and a thorough report is given.

Preoperative Care for Woman Having Cesarean Birth

Perioperative care starts with the admission assessment done for all patients admitted to the labor unit. A baseline FHR strip of 20 to 30 minutes is obtained and assessed for abnormalities. If labor has begun, the woman and fetus are monitored according to policy. The woman and family are told what to expect and questions are answered. The consent is signed by the woman and witnessed. Verification of nothing-by-mouth (NPO) status is made and IV access is obtained by venipuncture. Laboratory specimens are drawn if needed. A Foley catheter is inserted and any preoperative medications ordered are given. The abdomen is prepped according to policy. Family members who will attend the birth are gowned and prepped. When all is finished, the woman is taken to the operating room, assisted to the table, and assisted to a supine position with a wedge under one side.

Risk of Adverse Surgical Events During Cesarean Birth

Women who have a cesarean birth are at risk for **retained foreign bodies**. The risk is highest when the cesarean birth is unplanned and emergent. It is also increased in the obese woman. This can be prevented by doing sponge counts and counting instruments and needles. An x-ray can also be obtained before the patient leaves the table. The woman is also at risk for **anesthesia awareness** during general anesthesia. This includes an awareness of sounds and activity, and the feeling of paralysis, panic, helplessness, and pain. This experience can be mentally disturbing, and cause chronic post-traumatic stress disorder (PTSD) for years afterwards. Obstetric patients are at higher risk because of the light anesthesia given to spare the fetus. The Joint Commission has recommended that policies be put into place at each facility to deal with this complication.

Amnioinfusion

Amnioinfusion involves the infusion of room temperature normal saline or Ringer's lactate into the uterus through the cervix via an intrauterine pressure catheter. A bolus of 250 to 500 mL is infused over 20 to 30 minutes. A continuous infusion of 2 to 3 mL/min may then be given until variable decelerations resolve. Up to 1,000 mL may be infused. **Amnioinfusion** is performed when there are variable FHR decelerations during the first stage of labor when oligohydramnios is present. This alleviates cord compression. Its use in thick meconium staining has not been shown to prevent meconium aspiration syndrome or death, so it is not used for this indication.

Use of Forceps During Delivery

Forceps are used when the birth must be expedited for the sake of the mother or fetus. This may occur during a breech birth, or when the mother is compromised by cardiac or pulmonary disease, exhaustion, or regional analgesia. Macrosomia, occiput posterior presentations, fetal distress, advanced maternal age, and prolonged first or second stages of labor are other indications. Depending on criteria, **outlet, low, or midforceps** are used, and **piper forceps** are used in a breech delivery to deliver the head. The cervix must be completely dilated, membranes ruptured, and the fetal head must be engaged. Maternal analgesia is important. The woman should empty her bladder before forceps extraction is attempted. Injuries to both fetus and mother can result.

Criteria for Use of Outlet, Low, and Midforceps

Outlet forceps are used when the fetal head is visible at the vaginal opening. The labia are not separated. At this point, the skull is at the pelvic floor. The head is in a right or left occiput anterior or posterior position and rotation is not over 45 degrees. **Low forceps** are used when the fetal skull is at +2 station or more but has not yet reached the pelvic floor. Rotation is less than or greater than 45 degrees. **Midforceps** are used when there is engagement of the head in the pelvis but the station is above +2.

Vacuum Extraction

Vacuum extraction is performed instead of using forceps. A soft cup is placed on the fetal scalp and suction is applied to pull the fetus out of the birth canal. Up to three pulls may be attempted. No more than 600 mm Hg pressure is used. The total amount of time that the vacuum cup is applied should not exceed 15 to 20 minutes. It is not used for rotation. Up to 28% of fetuses develop a cephalohematoma after vacuum extraction is performed. Other fetal intracranial hemorrhages may result as well as scalp abrasions and lacerations. Maternal complications include vaginal and cervical lacerations, extended episiotomy, sphincter damage, bladder injury, hemorrhage, uterine atony, increased vaginal bleeding, anemia, and pain.

- 53 -

Pain Management

Origin of Pain During Labor

The acute pain of labor is affected by variations in the individual patient, past experience and perception of pain, and past and present obstetrical procedures. **Pain** is affected by the rate of dilatation, intensity and length of contractions, fetal position, and fetal size. The lack of sleep and exhaustion reduces pain tolerance as the labor progresses. The mother's age and past pregnancy and delivery experiences also influence her perception of labor pain. Physiologically, labor pain has its origin in uterine muscle hypoxia and the accumulation of lactic acid from uterine contractions. Pain also occurs with the stretching of the tissues in the lower uterine segment, cervix, ovaries, fallopian tubes, and uterine ligaments, and, later, the pelvic floor, vagina, vulva, and perineum. Bone pain from pressure on the bony pelvis or lower spine contributes to discomfort. Pressure on the bladder, urethra, and rectum cause pain during the second stage as well.

Sedative, Hypnotics, and Parenteral Analgesia to Control Labor Pain

Sedatives and hypnotics depress the CNS and provide relief from anxiety. They allow the woman to rest and conserve her energy for active labor and birth. They are given early in labor to decrease the neonatal effects. Barbiturates such as secobarbital and pentobarbital are used. H_1-receptor antagonists such as promethazine, hydroxyzine, and propiomazine hydrochloride are given along with narcotics to decrease nausea and vomiting, provide sedation, and relieve anxiety. Medications given **parenterally** to decrease labor pain include opioids, synthetic opioids, and opioid agonist-antagonists. These drugs affect different receptor sites on nerve cells in the CNS to control pain. Opioids used include morphine and meperidine. Meperidine has a long-lasting effect on neonatal behavior so its use during labor has decreased. Synthetic opioids such as fentanyl citrate and opioid agonist-antagonists such as butorphanol tartrate and nalbuphine hydrochloride are also used during labor. All of these medications are given when labor is well established because they decrease labor contraction frequency and duration and FHR variability. All can cause maternal respiratory depression and resultant fetal distress.

Control of Epidural Infusions During Second Stage of Labor

Epidural infusion used to be stopped during the second stage when the mother was unable to feel the urge to push or was pushing inadequately. This was done in the effort to shorten the second stage. When the woman labors pain free and then suddenly feels severe pain, a longer second stage or operative birth may then result. This is the opposite of the desired result. Instead of stopping the epidural infusion, **combine medications** to provide more analgesia and less motor blockage. The level of blockage and type and amount of medication infused should be analyzed and changed to provide the desired effect.

Laboring Down

Laboring down is the passive fetal descent that occurs when the woman has had regional analgesia/anesthesia and cannot feel the urge to push at full dilatation. Current trends are to allow 1 hour for multiparas or 2 hours for nulliparas for passive fetal descent to occur. This spontaneous descent causes far fewer FHR decelerations and less maternal fatigue, and results in fewer maternal urinary and pelvic floor injuries. When fetal descent stretches the muscles of the pelvic floor, the woman will feel the urge to push and birth will occur. She should push for as long as she is comfortable, and only when she feels the urge. Coach her to take several breaths between her pushing efforts.

- 54 -

Neuraxial Analgesia During Labor and Delivery

Neuraxial analgesia techniques, including epidurals, spinals, and combined epidural-spinal, have grown in popularity. This is because they have a flexibility and effectiveness that make them ideal for this purpose. They cause less depression of the maternal and fetal CNS. These methods of providing regional anesthesia require skill to provide effective analgesia while retaining as much motor control as possible. A catheter placed in the epidural space delivers an infusion that is intermittent, continuous, or patient-controlled. Local anesthetics used include bupivacaine, lidocaine, and ropivacaine. Narcotics such as fentanyl, sufentanil, alfentanil, and remifentanil are often added to the infusion to lessen the amount of anesthetic used and therefore decrease the amount of motor blockage. The duration and quality of pain relief is also improved.

Local Anesthetic or Pudendal Block During Second Stage of Labor

Local anesthetics such as lidocaine hydrochloride or chloroprocaine hydrochloride are used to numb the perineum and posterior vagina prior to an episiotomy. The anesthesia lasts 20 to 40 minutes and may need to be given again prior to the repair. A **pudendal block** uses the same **local anesthetics** injected into the pudendal nerve to numb the lower vagina, vulva, and perineum. The perineum is often injected also when a pudendal is used. There is a risk of hematoma or infection at the injection site. Inadvertent injection into a vein can cause hypotension, arrhythmias, and seizures so aspiration is performed prior to injection.

General Anesthesia in the Birth Process

General anesthesia is rarely used for vaginal birth but may be used for emergency procedures and Caesarean births if the mother is not a good candidate for epidural or subarachnoid block. Maternal complications can include aspiration of stomach contents, especially if the woman has not been NPO, and this can result in postoperative chemical pneumonitis. Therefore, an oral antacid is sometimes administered prior to anesthesia. A wedge should be placed under the woman's right hip to displace the uterus to the left prior to administration of anesthesia. The woman may experience respiratory depression, and this can affect the oxygenation of the fetus. **General anesthesia** can also result in relaxation of the uterine muscles, and if this persists in the postoperative period, it increases the risk of postpartum hemorrhage. General anesthesia is contraindicated with a high risk or preterm fetus because of fetal depression. Anesthesia usually affects the fetus within 2 minutes, so rapid delivery reduces risks to the fetus.

Nonpharmacologic Pain Management

Nonpharmacologic pain strategies include controlling pain using cutaneous, auditory, visual, and cognitive methods. **Cutaneous methods** include the use of touch, massage, back rubs, and counterpressure. Also included are the use of hydrotherapy and the application of heat or cold. Maternal movement and positioning is encouraged. Acupuncture or acupressure may also be employed. **Auditory and visual methods** include focusing on an object, and the use of distraction, hypnosis, music, and breathing techniques to reduce pain. This helps to prevent the transmission of pain sensations to the central nervous system. **Cognitive methods** help to control interpretation of pain. These methods employ education about pain and the importance of relaxation. Imagery may be used. Constant support during labor is also part of cognitive pain control.

- 55 -

Non-Pharmacologic Methods of Pain Management During Labor and Delivery

Positioning and Progressive Relaxation

Comfort measures during labor/delivery include:

- **Positioning**: Assist to turn at least every hour or to sit in a warm shower or rocking chair to increase relaxation and relieve discomfort. If in bed, body, arms, and legs should be supported comfortably with pillows or bolsters with joints slightly flexed. If supine, the head of the bed should be elevated to at least 30° and support placed under the right side to tilt abdomen to the left to relieve uterine pressure on the vena cava.
- **Progressive relaxation**: Helps relax muscles and relieve tension so that uterine contractions are more effective. Progressive relaxation involves first tightening muscles and holding the tension for a few seconds and then relaxing them, concentrating on the difference in feeling between the tense and relaxed muscle states and imagining the tension flowing out of the muscles. Relaxation is usually done bilaterally, starting with the feet and moving upward through the muscles of the lower legs, the hands, the lower arms, the upper arms and finally the abdomen and chest, the neck, and the face.

Prepared Childbirth

Prepared childbirth is an approach in which the mother and partner/spouse are educated about pregnancy, labor, and delivery. Popular methods of prepared childbirth include:

- The **Lamaze method** encourages women to take control of their bodies and utilizes various techniques (dissociation relaxation, relaxation exercises, and breathing patterns) to alleviate discomfort and facilitate birth. Lamaze teaches that birth is a natural process that should be as free of interventions/medications as possible.
- The **Kitzinger (psychosexual) method** encourages women to take an active part in the birthing process, which is viewed as very natural. Kitzinger encourages alternatives to the usual hospital birthing procedures, including home births, birth rooms, and water births. Women learn chest breathing combined with abdominal relaxation, touch relaxation, and visualization.
- The **Bradley method** of natural childbirth is usually taught in a series of 12 weekly classes in which the pregnant woman and her partner participate with a goal of natural childbirth without the use of drugs, Caesarean, or episiotomy to ensure both the mother and infant are healthy.

Labor Coach and Patterned Breathing

Comfort measures during labor/delivery include:

- **Labor coach**: Assists the woman by providing support, guidance, and advocacy. The coach encourages the woman, uses measures (such as massage) to reduce discomfort, provides distraction, and assists the woman to utilize breathing patterns to reduce discomfort. The coach should remain calm and speak softly, use a gentle touch, and move slowly to help the woman relax.

- 56 -

- **Patterned breathing**: Slow deep breathing is done while focusing on relaxing different parts of the breathing to relieve discomfort of contractions. Rapid mouth breathing (1 per second) is used during contractions in the active stage of labor. Variable breathing (hee-hee-hoo) is used during the first stage of labor if the woman is especially tense or tired. Expulsion breathing (taking a deep breath and then holding the breath while leaning forward and pushing) is used during stage two of labor to help move the fetus down the birth canal.

Obstetric Complications

Labor and Placental Disorders

Interventions for Shoulder Dystocia

During a birth with shoulder dystocia, action must be taken to deliver the body within 5 minutes if at all possible. The risk of neonatal acidemia rises greatly if it takes longer. At the first sign of **shoulder dystocia**, the woman is placed in a knee-chest position while supine (McRoberts maneuver). This maneuver changes the angle of the maternal pelvis to the lumbar spine, causing a flattening of the sacrum. These changes may ease delivery. If not, suprapubic pressure is applied in an attempt to dislodge the impacted shoulder as the head is directed downwards. If these interventions do not work immediately then it is prudent to call for help. Extra personnel will be needed to position the mother's legs and to prepare to resuscitate the newborn if needed. Other maneuvers that may be attempted include the Woods, Schwartz-Dixon, and Gaskin maneuvers. If the fetus is unable to be delivered vaginally, the Zavanelli maneuver of cephalic replacement back into the vagina and a cesarean birth may be performed.

Uterine Dysfunction During Labor

Uterine dysfunction can be caused by epidural analgesia, chorioamnionitis, and maternal position during labor, pushing, and delivery. There are 2 types of uterine dysfunction as defined by ACOG:

- **Protraction disorders** are those in which dilatation or descent take longer than normal. Protracted dilatation is that which occurs at a rate that is less than 1.2 cm/h in the nullipara and less than 1.5 cm/h in the multipara. Protracted descent occurs at less than 1 cm/h in the nullipara and less than 2 cm/h in the multipara.
- **Arrest disorders** are those in which dilatation or descent stop progressing. Arrested dilatation is diagnosed after 2 hours without dilatation in the nullipara and 1 hour in the multipara. Arrested descent is considered to be lack of descent for 1 hour in either nullipara or multipara.

Fetopelvic Disproportion

Fetopelvic disproportion means that either the fetus is too big or the pelvis is too small. Digital examination, MRI, CT scans, and X-ray pelvimetry are tools used to help estimate pelvic capacity. No specific fetal size can be blamed because each maternal pelvis has its own limit. Abnormal presentations contribute to fetopelvic disproportion. Fetal hydrocephalus also causes difficulty. Pelvic contraction may be one of the following types or a combination:

- **Pelvic inlet contraction**: The pelvic inlet should measure 10 cm or more at its shortest anteroposterior diameter and 12 cm or more at its greatest transverse diameter. The normal diagonal conjugate is 11.5 or more. A smaller pelvic inlet is contracted.
- **Midpelvis contraction**: Interischial spinous diameter should be over 10 cm. Midpelvic contraction can be inferred when spines are prominent, the sacrosciatic notch is narrow, or the pelvic side-walls converge.
- **Pelvic outlet contraction**: The interischial tuberous diameter should be over 8 cm.

- 58 -

Dystocia

Dystocia is abnormal labor caused by problems with the power of contractions and pushing, problems with the passenger or fetus, or problems within the passageway or pelvis. Three types of abnormalities can occur to cause **dystocia**:

- **Abnormal power**: Uterine contractions that are not adequate enough to cause dilatation and effacement because of lack of coordination or intensity, or ineffectiveness of the mother's pushing efforts.
- **Abnormal passenger**: Fetal problems that cause dystocia include malpresentation, position, or abnormal development of the fetus.
- **Abnormal passageway**: Contraction of the bony pelvis and soft tissue abnormalities that hinder birth.

Precipitous Labor and Delivery

Labor that takes less than 3 hours from start to birth of the baby is **precipitous**. Dilatation can occur at a rate of 5 cm/h in the nullipara and 10 cm/h in the multipara. Precipitous labor and delivery occurs as a result of abnormally low soft tissue resistance in the passageway. It is also a result of abnormally intense contractions of the uterus and abdominal muscles. Contractions often occur less than 2 minutes apart during the entire labor. Complications from precipitous labor and delivery can include placental abruption and postpartum hemorrhage from a hypotonic uterus. If the mother is a multipara and tissues of the vagina and perineum are compliant, there may be no lacerations or tears. Noncompliance of these structures can result in uterine rupture or tissue lacerations. Neonatal complications can include acidemia, meconium staining, low Apgar scores, Erb's or Duchenne brachial palsy, intracranial injury, and birth injuries.

Placenta Previa

Placenta previa is the presence of the placenta over the cervical os. A **marginal placenta previa** is one in which the edge of the placenta is within 2 to 3 cm of the cervical os. The edge of the placenta must be farther than 2 to 3 cm for normal delivery and no increased risk for intrapartum hemorrhage. Symptoms often occur for the first time in the second or third trimester when uterine bleeding occurs. Bleeding may not occur until labor begins. Bleeding from placenta previa may be intermittent or continuous. Bleeding may be affected by uterine activity. Hemorrhage and maternal and fetal distress may occur. A cesarean birth must be a readily available emergency option during labor and vaginal birth with a placenta previa. Mothers older than 35 years of age are at higher risk for placenta previa. Those with scarring of the uterus, uterine fibroids, endometritis, or uterine anomalies are also at greater risk. Cigarette smoking, multiparity, multiple gestations, large placenta, and fetal hydrops fetalis contribute to the risk as well.

Abnormal Placental Implantation

Defective decidua basalis is thought to be the cause of **abnormal adherence of the placenta to the uterine wall**. This is more common when there has been a previous cesarean section or when placenta previa is present. It is diagnosed when manual removal of the placenta fails and surgical intervention is performed. There is a high risk of maternal hemorrhage and hysterectomy may be necessary. Three varieties are recognized:

- **Placenta accreta**: The decidual basalis is absent so the placenta grows directly into the myometrium of the uterine wall. Only a portion or all of the placenta's cotyledons may be adherent to the uterine wall in this way. This is the most common variety.

- 59 -

- **Placenta increta**: Trophoblastic cells invade the myometrium of the uterine wall.
- **Placenta percreta**: Trophoblastic cells penetrate through the uterine wall and invade other organs in the vicinity such as the bladder.

Uterine Rupture and Dehiscence

The uterine wall may **separate** at the site of a previous scar. If the fetal membranes stay intact and the fetus stays in the uterus, a dehiscence has occurred. When the uterine wall **ruptures** and part or the entire fetus extrudes into the peritoneal cavity, death can quickly occur in the fetus and mother without rapid cesarean section. Symptoms of both can include sharp, tearing uterine pain, FHR decelerations, vomiting, fainting, vaginal bleeding, tachycardia, hypotension, and shock. Factors associated with uterine rupture include uterine hyperstimulation, previous uterine surgery, use of prostaglandins, multiparity, abdominal traumatic injury, and fundal pressure.

Uterine Inversion

Inversion is the turning inside out of the uterus. It can be caused by fundal pressure and traction on the umbilical cord. It can also occur during uterine atony, with large fetuses or short umbilical cords, from adherent placental tissues, and from the use of oxytocin. It can also occur spontaneously without obvious cause. Sometimes only the fundus inverts (partial inversion) and other times the fundus protrudes through the cervical opening (complete inversion). **Inversion** may be *visualized* or *occult*. There is sudden severe pelvic pain, hemorrhage, and hypotension. There will be a firm mass below the cervix felt by bimanual exam. The uterus must be immediately replaced manually prior to delivery of the placenta. Tocolytics or general anesthesia may be required to do this. IV fluids and blood are given to replace blood loss as needed. Antibiotics and a nasogastric tube may also be needed.

Vasa Previa

Vasa previa is an abnormality where at least one of the fetal blood vessels lies across the internal cervical os. The fetal umbilical vein and arteries lie unprotected on the membrane wall on their way to the placenta. This predisposes the fetus to hemorrhage if one of the vessels is injured during membrane rupture that occurs spontaneously or artificially. The FHR reacts immediately to the vessel damage and death occurs in 56% of all cases. An immediate cesarean section is indicated. Diagnosis may be made prenatally by transvaginal Doppler ultrasound or routine ultrasound that examines placental cord insertion. A planned cesarean increases the fetal survival rate to 97%.

Abruptio Placentae

Abruptio placenta is the detachment of the placenta from the uterine wall. This causes a hemorrhage that may flow out of the uterus or that may be concealed within the uterus. The presence of sudden, intense uterine pain and bright red bloody vaginal drainage alerts the nurse to the abruptio. A concealed hemorrhage may cause symptoms of sudden uterine pain, hypertonus, and fetal tachycardia or bradycardia, absent variability, late decelerations, or a sinusoidal FHR pattern. When an **abruptio placenta** is suspected, a Kleihauer-Betke test may be done to detect fetal blood cells in the maternal circulation or in a vaginal bleeding specimen. If the abruption is small and the maternal-fetal status is stable, then the woman is observed until she reaches term and spontaneous labor occurs. On the other end of the spectrum, a large abruption will prompt an emergency cesarean section. The woman is at risk for disseminated intravascular coagulation (DIC) from the release of thromboplastin from the placental site into her bloodstream during abruptio placenta.

Complications Associated with Rupture of Membranes Prior to Labor Initiation

Spontaneous rupture of membranes that occurs without the presence of uterine contractions occurs in 8% of women with term pregnancies. The preferred method of management includes induction with oxytocin if labor does not begin in 6 to 12 hours. This results in fewer intrapartum and postpartum infections. Women who are sent home with ruptured membranes and no labor have a higher rate of infections than when they are kept in the hospital and induced. **Rupture of membranes** without signs of labor happens more frequently in black women.

Brow Presentation

Brow presentation is characterized by presentation of the fetal brow (area on the face from the orbital ridge to the anterior fontanel) at the pelvic inlet. It is rare. Engagement and delivery are impossible unless the head is very small or the pelvis very large. This presentation has the same causes as face presentation: anencephaly, nuchal umbilical cord loops, large fetus, and pelvic contraction. **Brow presentation** may change to a face or occiput presentation to allow vaginal birth to occur. Caput succedaneum occurs over the forehead and may be extensive, deforming the face.

Transverse Lie Presentation

This presentation occurs when the fetus is lying across the maternal pelvis. If the fetal-maternal axis is less then perpendicular, an oblique lie is present. The oblique lie turns into perpendicular when labor begins. The fetal shoulder is usually over the pelvic inlet with the head in one maternal iliac fossa and the breech in the opposite fossa. The fetal back may be anterior or posterior. Causes of **transverse lie** include parity of 4 pregnancies or more, relaxed abdominal wall and pendulous abdomen, placenta previa, pelvic contraction, prematurity, uterine abnormalities, and polyhydramnios.

Compound Presentation

Compound presentations are a complication in which a *fetal extremity* presents alongside the presenting part. A hand or arm may be positioned next to the head. A breech delivery may be complicated by a hand. Rarely, one or both legs may present next to the head. Compound presentations are more common in preterm births. The extra presenting part may not interfere with labor. It may move out of the way as the main presenting part descends. An arm presenting along with the head may prevent descent and have to be pushed up and out of the way. The extremity may suffer ischemic damage from pressure during labor and birth.

Persistent Occiput Transverse Position

This position is usually a transition into the occiput anterior position and is temporary. If uterine contractions are weak as a result of analgesia, rotation may slow. Oxytocin may be infused in this case to increase contractions enough to complete spontaneous rotation. Outlet forceps may be required to rotate the head to an **anterior** or **posterior** presentation for delivery. There may be a lot of molding and caput formation of the fetal head and forceps must be used without extreme force. When the maternal pelvis is platypelloid or android shaped, the fetal head may fail to engage, resulting in the need for a cesarean birth.

Face Presentation

Face presentation is when the fetal neck is hyperextended and the chin is presenting. The occiput is pressing against the fetal back. The chin may be anterior or posterior relative to the maternal

- 61 -

pelvis. When it is posterior, the fetal brow is against the maternal symphysis pubis and further descent cannot occur. This position may convert spontaneously to anterior and allow fetal neck flexion and birth. This presentation occurs frequently when an anencephalic fetus is present. It also occurs more if there are loops of umbilical cord around the fetal neck and when pelvic contractions are present or the fetus is large. Multiparous women with or without pendulous abdomens are more prone.

Breech Presentations

Breech presentations may be one of three types:

- **Frank breech**: The fetal legs are flexed at the hips and extended at the knees, bringing the feet close to the head.
- **Complete breech**: Both legs are flexed at the hips and knees and the legs are wrapped around the body.
- **Incomplete breech**: One or both legs are extended at the hip. A foot or knee is then the presenting part. Both feet and knees may present.

Factors associated with breech presentations include polyhydramnios, oligohydramnios, anencephaly, hydrocephaly, relaxation of uterine muscles due to increased parity, multiple gestation, uterine anomalies, pelvic tumors, and previous breech deliveries. The place of placental implantation may be a factor with the cornual-fundal site seen more often with breech deliveries.

Breech Delivery

Since the umbilical cord is compressed during a **breech delivery**, delivery of the entire body must quickly follow the breech. The head is molded as it enters the birth canal after the breech is born. This sometimes takes a few minutes during which the fetus may suffer asphyxia. The use of forceps to deliver the head expedites birth but can cause trauma to the fetal head and vaginal canal. In the case of preterm birth, the much smaller body of the fetus may be delivered before the cervix is dilated enough for the head to pass. Cervical incisions may be required to deliver the head without delay. Breech delivery complicated by the fetal arm around the neck can be deadly. Cord complications occur frequently with breech presentations and can complicate delivery. Breech deliveries should be well staffed and equipped to handle resuscitation of the newborn and maternal analgesia.

Persistent Occiput Posterior Presentation

When the head presents in the occiput posterior position, it often rotates to the anterior position spontaneously. It is not able to rotate when the midpelvis is narrow in the transverse plane. In most cases, vaginal delivery can be accomplished. Forceps may be needed when the **occiput** is directly **posterior**. They may also be used to rotate to the anterior position. Sometimes manual rotation is able to turn to the anterior position for delivery. An episiotomy is usually needed to complete delivery. The woman will need more analgesia than just a local for this type of delivery. Cesarean birth may be needed in some cases.

Vaginal Abnormalities That Can Impact Delivery

Vaginal abnormalities do not usually affect delivery unless they directly obstruct the birth canal. Vaginal abnormalities may include:

- **Double vagina**: A true double vagina has 2 distinctly separate vaginas, each ending with its own cervix. Sometimes one passage ends in a wall rather than a second cervix.
- **Atresia**: Atresia of the vagina may be partial or complete and is often due to Rokitansky-Kuster-Hauser syndrome or androgen insensitivity syndrome.
- **Transversely septate vagina**: This anomaly includes a septum that forms across the birth canal.
- **Longitudinally septate vagina**: A septum runs the length of the birth canal. It can be confused with a double vagina.

Uterine Malformations That Can Affect Pregnancy

Anomalies of the uterus include:

- **Segmental hypoplasia or agenesis**: Inadequate development or absence of the fallopian tubes, fundus, cervix, vagina, or combination.
- **Unicornuate uterus**: The upper half of one side of the uterus that connects with a fallopian tube is partially or totally missing, may be represented by a horn that may or may not communicate with the uterus.
- **Uterine didelphys**: The normal uterus is divided through the center so there are 2 smaller uteruses with their own cervix, each attached to 1 fallopian tube.
- **Bicornuate uterus**: The fundus is indented into the uterine cavity. This indent can extend the entire way down through the cavity to just above the cervix, dividing the uterus into 2 cavities that communicate.
- **Septate uterus**: A septum develops, partially or completely separating the uterus into 2 cavities.
- **Arcuate**: There is a slight indentation of the fundus into the uterine cavity.
- **Diethylstilbestrol-induced anomalies**: Exposed daughters have a high risk of vaginal and cervical cancer and reproductive tract anomalies.

Cervical Abnormalities That Can Affect Delivery

Several conditions can have an effect on delivery. Vulvar edema can be present throughout pregnancy or there may be infectious or inflammatory lesions in the perineal area that interfere with episiotomy and repair. Large cysts of the Bartholin glands can interfere with delivery and may have to be aspirated. Extensive venereal warts (condyloma acuminata) may make a cesarean birth necessary. Genital mutilation that partially closes the vaginal opening will require surgical excision of the scar tissue or cesarean section if the woman prefers. Active genital herpes infection will also make a cesarean birth necessary.

The different types of **cervical abnormalities** can include:

- **Double cervix**: There are 2 distinct cervixes. A longitudinally septate vagina is frequently present as well.
- **Atresia**: The absence of a cervix, providing an effective barrier to conception. Frequently associated with other uterine and vaginal abnormalities.

- 63 -

- **Septate cervix**: There is a septum through the center of the cervix. Frequently associated with a uterine or vaginal septum.
- **Single hemicervix**: Half of the cervix is present.
- **Cervical stenosis**: Caused by cervical trauma. Usually softens during labor but may not dilate, making cesarean birth necessary.

Velamentous Cord Insertion

Velamentous cord insertion is an abnormality in which the cord inserts into the membranes rather than the middle of the placenta, traveling through the chorion and amnion to reach the placental margin, leaving exposed vessels unprotected by Wharton's jelly. This can cause shearing of the blood vessels during delivery, leading to hemorrhage. Additionally, the exposed vessels are vulnerable to compression, which can result in fetal anoxia. **Velamentous cord insertion** is most common with placenta previa and multiple gestations. While incidence is only about 1% for singletons, the incidence increases to almost 9% with twins, so the nurse must be alert for indications. Velamentous cord insertion is associated with about 25% of spontaneous abortions. Velamentous cord insertion may result in vasa previa if the velamentous vessels are lower than the presenting part because they may rupture, causing the fetus to exsanguinate, especially during onset of labor or amniotomy. Indications of velamentous cord insertion include excessive bleeding and fetal distress. Treatment includes careful monitoring and Caesarean.

Prolapsed Cord

A prolapse of the umbilical cord occurs when the umbilical cord precedes the fetus in the birth canal and becomes entrapped by the descending fetus. An **occult cord prolapse** occurs when the umbilical cord is beside or just ahead of the fetal head. About half of prolapses occur in the second stage of labor and relate to premature delivery, multiple gestation, polyhydramnios, breech delivery, and an excessively long umbilical cord. Some cases are precipitated by obstetric interventions, such as amniotomy, external version, and application of scalp electrode for monitoring. As contractions occur and the head descends, this applies pressure to the umbilical cord, occluding blood flow and causing hypoxia and bradycardia. The decrease in blood flow through the umbilical vessels can cause impaired gas exchange, and if pressure on the cord is not relieved, the fetus can suffer severe neurological damage or death. Management includes elevating the presenting part off the cord, having the mother elevate her knees to the chest, and preparing for Caesarean.

Amniotic Fluid Embolism

Amniotic fluid embolism (AKA anaphylactoid syndrome of pregnancy) occurs when amniotic fluid enters the mother's circulatory system, such as may occur during Caesareans and labor and delivery, during which small tears in the lower uterine segment or cervix allow amniotic fluid to enter maternal circulation. In most mothers, this poses no problem, but some mothers have an anaphylactoid response that can include hypotension, pulmonary edema, cyanosis, coagulopathy, dyspnea, seizures, and cardiac arrest for the mother as well as fetal distress. The *initial phase* usually includes cardiovascular collapse with severe pulmonary vasoconstriction, which results in inability of the heart to transfer blood from the right to the left and marked oxygen desaturation with neurological injury. Uterine hypertonus and lack of blood flow to the uterus occurs. The *second phase*, if the mother survives the first, usually includes lung injury and coagulopathy. Treatment includes immediate CPR, circulatory support, and blood and blood components as needed. If undelivered, emergent delivery is critical to save the infant.

Chorioamnionitis

Chorioamnionitis is inflammation of fetal membranes (amniotic sac) usually by viral or bacterial infection, most commonly associated with premature rupture of membranes, which allows pathogens to migrate through the cervix and into the uterus. **Chorioamnionitis** from ascending pathogens, such as *N. gonorrhoeae,* may also trigger premature rupture of membranes. The chorion is initially infected and the tissue adjacent to the cervical os. As the infection progresses, it involves the full-thickness of the membranes, spreading along the surface and infecting the amniotic fluid and the umbilical cord (funisitis). The fetus may become infected through blood, aspiration, swallowing, or direct contact with the infected amniotic fluid, and fetal sepsis may occur. Indications of chorioamnionitis include fever above 38° C/100.4° F, uterine tenderness, and maternal and fetal tachycardia. The mother's white blood cell count may be elevated. Purulent vaginal discharge occurs late. Treatment includes cultures, antibiotics, and steroid therapy. Immediate delivery/Caesarean is indicated although labor may begin spontaneously.

Effects of Obesity on Labor Process, Fetus, and Newborn

A pregnant woman is considered obese with weight 50% greater than ideal weight, weight greater than 200 lb. (91 kg), or BMI greater than 29. The woman is at increased risk of developing **gestational diabetes mellitus** and **hypertension**. The second stage of labor is often prolonged because the myometrium is overstretched. Additionally, labor is difficult and associated with macrosomia and shoulder dystocia, which can cause permanent brachial plexus injury in the newborn. Because of excessive fatty tissue in the abdomen, monitoring of fetal heart rate and contractions may be difficult. During labor and delivery, the woman is at increased risk of uterine rupture and lacerations. The obese pregnant woman is more likely to require Caesarean but is at risk for excessive blood loss during surgery (>1000 mL), difficulty with intubation, and prolonged operative time as well as the need for hysterectomy. Postoperatively, the woman is at greater risk of complications (DVT and infection).

Intrapartal and Post-Partal Hemorrhage

Intrapartal hemorrhage often occurs because of placenta previa or abruptio placentae or disseminated intravascular coagulation (which may be triggered by release of tissue thromboplastin with abruptio placentae or with a dead fetus). **Post-partal hemorrhage** is blood loss greater than 500 mL following vaginal birth or greater than 1000 mL following Caesarean, or saturation of more than one peri-pad in 15 minutes. A drop in hematocrit of 10% or more may also indicate hemorrhage but may not be accurate with hemorrhage. Hemorrhage:

- **Early postpartum**: Occurs within 24 hours of childbirth and up to 90% is caused by uterine atony, which is often associated with overdistention (multiple gestations, large infant, hydramnios) or weak muscles (multiparity). Induced or precipitous labor increases risk. Early hemorrhage may also be caused by trauma (lacerations and hematomas).
- **Late postpartum**: Occurs more than 24 hours (often up to 6 to 14 days) after childbirth and usually results from subinvolution of uterus or retained placental fragments.

Following delivery, the nurse must monitor the woman carefully for increased bleeding, severe pain, tachycardia, and uncontracted uterus, as these signs may indicate **postpartal hemorrhage**. The nurse must massage the fundus and apply firm but gentle fundal pressure only to the contracted uterus to express clots as applying pressure to an uncontracted uterus may result in increased hemorrhage and uterine inversion. The nurse should also relieve a distended bladder, which can prevent uterine contraction. The patient may need IV oxytocin or bimanual compression

- 65 -

of the uterus to control bleeding. If bleeding is caused by trauma, surgical repair is needed. **Balloon tamponade** may be needed to control bleeding. Specially designed catheters have a balloon (usually 500 mL capacity) that is inflated with NS after insertion into the uterus. Many balloon catheters are bi-luminal so that blood can drain and be measured to determine if the pressure applied by the balloon is controlling bleeding. The balloon catheter should control bleeding within 5 to 15 minutes.

Preterm Labor

Preterm Labor

Preterm labor is uterine contractions causing cervical dilatation of more than 1 cm or effacement of 80% that occurs after 20 weeks and before 36 weeks of gestation. Uterine irritability is not **preterm labor** but should be monitored in case it turns into labor. The rate of preterm births prior to 37 weeks has risen 49% since 1982 to a 2006 rate of 12.7%. Most of the births occur at 34 to 36 weeks. The rise in the preterm birth rate has been attributed to the following: infertility treatments producing multiples, more mothers older than 35 years of age, higher incidence of medically induced prematurity, repeat cesareans prior to 37 weeks, advances in maternal and neonatal care that have allowed physicians to consider earlier births for maternal and fetal welfare, and an increased rate of fetal complications such as intrauterine growth restriction.

Cervical Length Measurements and Fetal Fibronectin Screening to Predict Preterm Birth

Cervical length can be measured by the use of ultrasound. Some preterm labor has been predicted by a cervical length of less than 30 mm. The method has been 24% accurate and is not helpful in preventing preterm birth at this time. **Fetal fibronectin** is a biochemical marker produced in the decidua of the uterus. It is a substance that helps form the bond at the uteroplacental junction. It is not present normally in vaginal secretions until after 36 weeks of gestation. Its presence prior to that at a level of greater than 50 ng/mL predicts preterm labor. Tests for fetal fibronectin must be done correctly. The woman must abstain from sex for 24 hours prior to the test. Cervical exams must be delayed for the same amount of time. Douches must not be used and there should be no vaginal bleeding or infections of the vagina or amniotic sac present when the specimen is taken.

Genetic Risk Factors for Preterm Birth

Studies continue to discover the influence of genetics on the rate of preterm birth. They have shown that women who smoke and have a certain gene change are more prone to intrauterine growth retardation and preterm birth. Women who were themselves born prematurely are also more likely to give birth prematurely. Ongoing studies are examining certain genes to see if they may play a role in preterm birth. Proinflammatory cytokines that are involved in infections and premature rupture of membranes are areas of study. Vasculopathic genes involved in preeclampsia and other vascular problems and the labor cascade genes that initiate labor are also being studied.

Risk Factors for Preterm Birth

There are many risk factors for preterm birth. The 3 most common are *multiple pregnancies*, a *previous preterm birth*, and *uterine or cervical abnormalities*. Other risk factors include medical problems with the current pregnancy such as too short of an interval between pregnancies, problems with the fetus, vaginal bleeding, periodontal disease, infection, and premature rupture of membranes. Pregnancy conditions such as obesity, diabetes mellitus, hypertension, clotting problems, or mothers with a low prepregnancy weight contribute to the risk status. Black mothers, mothers who are younger than 17 or older than 35 years of age, or those of low socioeconomic status are at higher risk. The lack of prenatal care and high-risk behaviors such as smoking, drinking, and drug use are risk factors. The presence of stress, domestic violence, long work hours, or long hours on her feet will put the mother at risk for preterm birth as well.

Antibiotic Administration to Women with Preterm Labor

The CDC and ACOG recommend **vaginal and rectal group B streptococcal screening cultures** for all pregnant women at 35 to 37 weeks' gestation, and the administration of antibiotics for treatment of group B streptococcus (GBS) under the following conditions:

- presence of a positive GBS screening culture and plans for vaginal birth
- previous infant with invasive GBS infection
- GBS in urinary tract during pregnancy
- unknown GBS status and presence of ruptured membranes over 18 hours, delivery at less than 37 weeks' gestation, or maternal fever over 100.4 degrees Fahrenheit.

Antibiotics used include: penicillin G, ampicillin, cefazolin, clindamycin, erythromycin, and vancomycin.

Use of Tocolytics for Preterm Labor

Tocolytics are now most often used to delay preterm birth for 24 to 48 hours to allow glucocorticoids administered to the mother to have time to help fetal lungs mature. They are not advised as maintenance treatment or repeated treatment to stop preterm labor. The **tocolytic** used depends on the woman's state of health. Both fetus and mother are subject to major side effects, including maternal and fetal cardiac problems and maternal pulmonary edema. Beta-mimetic agents, magnesium sulfate, and indomethacin are used. Tocolytics should not be used in the presence of fetal distress or demise, infections within the amniotic sac, eclampsia, preeclampsia, or maternal cardiac instability.

Interventions for Preterm Labor

Women with preterm labor may use a **home uterine activity monitor**. The woman wears a tocodynamometer that monitors uterine activity. The information is then transmitted by telephone to the health care provider for interpretation. This method enables the early identification of subtle contractions that are not felt by the woman but can precede more frequent contractions leading to active labor. This intervention is expensive and not widely recommended for use by ACOG. **Bedrest** is most often recommended when preterm labor threatens. It has not been proven to work. Bedrest over 3 days in length results in loss of calcium and muscle tone, and glucose intolerance. Longer periods of bedrest cause constipation, fatigue, anxiety, depression, and bone demineralization. Mothers lose weight and infant birth weight declines. Bedrest also has a high impact on the family and finances. There are more maternal physical and emotional symptoms in the postpartum period. The nurse should be prepared to help the patient cope with family problems and find diversionary activity for the woman in bed.

Antenatal Glucocorticoids

Antenatal glucocorticoids prevent respiratory distress syndrome complications in the premature infant. They are given to women with signs of preterm labor between weeks 24 and 34. Either betamethasone or dexamethasone is given. Tocolytics may then be employed to delay birth for 24 to 48 hours to give the glucocorticoid time to help the fetal lungs mature. Betamethasone is given

- 67 -

in a dosage of 12 mg IM every 24 hours x 2 doses. Dexamethasone is given in a dosage of 6 mg IM every 12 hours x 2 doses. The effects last for 1 week. Further dosages are not advised at this time.

Multiple Gestation

Incidence of Multiple Gestations in the US

Multiple gestations are at an all-time record level in the United States. They account for 3.3% of all live births. The rate of twin births alone rose 70% from 1980 to 2004. The number of quadruplets or more doubled from 1989 to 2004. **Multiple births** are rising in the older maternal group since more women are delaying childbirth until later in life. Twins occur slightly more often among white women than black women. Higher order multiple pregnancies occur at a far higher rate in white women than in other women. The use of infertility treatments and assisted reproductive technologies has been the largest contributor to the rising rate of multiple gestations.

Physiological Aspects of Twinning

There are two types of twins. **Monozygotic twins** come from the same fertilized ovum and are identical. **Dizygotic twins** come from two fertilized ovum, are not identical, and may be of different sexes. Of the total number of twin pregnancies, one-third will be monozygotic and two-thirds dizygotic. Monozygotic twins may share a placenta (monochorionic) or have separate placentas (dichorionic). They may also share the same amniotic sac (monoamniotic) or have separate sacs (diamniotic). They are monochorionic and diamniotic 70% of the time. The sharing of placentas and amniotic sacs differs depending on which day the zygote divides into two. Dizygotic twins are always dichorionic and diamniotic.

Guidelines Affecting Assisted Reproductive Technology

Fertility-assisted pregnancies have a higher risk of poor outcomes when one fetus is involved. When twins are conceived with assisted reproduction, the outcome is better than of those conceived naturally. The concern lies with pregnancies with more than 2 fetuses. High-order multiples have a higher risk of preterm birth, low birth weight, and a higher mortality rate. There is also higher maternal morbidity and mortality with these pregnancies. The Society for Assisted Reproductive Technology (SART) and the American Society for Reproductive Medicine (ASRM) have recommended that the number of embryos transferred depends on the age of the mother. Mothers younger than 35 years of age should have 1 embryo transferred, mothers 35 to 37 should have 2, women 38 to 40 should have no more than 3, and women older than 40 should have no more than 5. These guidelines take into account the higher rate of pregnancy loss with increasing maternal age. The woman's medical condition, prognosis, and other individual circumstances also play a part in deciding how many embryos to transfer.

Multifetal Pregnancy Reduction

When a multifetal pregnancy is diagnosed after ovulation induction or assisted reproductive technology, the parents are offered the choice of reducing the number of fetuses carried to lower morbidity and mortality for the mother and the remaining fetuses. The procedure is done late in the first trimester. Fetuses with anomalies are selected first, normal fetuses second. An injection of potassium chloride into the thoracic cavity of the fetus is done to terminate. This procedure is not taken lightly by parents and may cause grief, stress, trauma, pain, and confusion. Emotional pain, sadness, and guilt are felt by women and may affect bonding with remaining babies after birth.

Labor with Multiples vs. Singleton Labor

Studies have been done concerning the **length of labor** with twins and triplets versus a single fetus. In studies concerning nulliparous women with twins versus nulliparous women with 1 fetus, the time taken to dilate from 4 to 10 cm was shorter for the twin labor. There was no difference in time for women who were multiparous. Similar results were found with triplet labors being shorter than singleton labor. Labor time is affected by presentation, birth weight, and use of analgesia/anesthesia in all cases. The length of the second stage of labor was not affected by multiples.

Delayed-Interval Birth

Delayed-interval birth occurs when there is an interval between the birth of 1 or more very premature infants and the remaining infant(s) in the uterus. Birth is delayed for the others in the hopes of improved survival. The interval averages from 6 to 31 days, with a case of 153 days reported. Benefits to perinatal or infant mortality depend on gestation and length of interval. Methods used to delay birth include the use of cervical cerclage, tocolytics, antibiotics, and corticosteroids. Intrauterine infection and maternal sepsis are complications for the mother. There are no study results about long-term infant morbidities.

Prolonged Pregnancy

Postterm Pregnancy

ACOG defines a postterm or **prolonged** pregnancy as one that has completed 42 weeks since the first day of the last menstrual period. The neonate will look postmature with deep creases, dry, wrinkled skin that peels, long nails, and an alert appearance. The neonate often shows evidence of weight loss and has a long, thin appearance. Due dates can be in error and a pregnancy may be less advanced than it is thought to be. A postterm pregnancy is likely to be repeated in subsequent pregnancies and is seen in families as influenced by the maternal genes. Fetal-placental factors may also play a role in prolongation of pregnancy.

Fetal and Neonatal Complications

A **post-term/prolonged pregnancy** lasts 294 days, or more than 42 weeks gestation. Post-term/prolonged pregnancy increases maternal risk of trauma, hemorrhage, prolonged labor, infection, and Caesarean. The placenta weakens after 40 weeks gestation, and oxygen and nutrients to the fetus may decrease, resulting in periods of hypoxia. Complications include macrosomia, shoulder dystocia, oligohydramnios, meconium aspiration, fetal distress, and stillbirths. Neonates may experience asphyxia, respiratory distress, polycythemia (in response to hypoxia), hypoglycemia, and dysmaturity syndrome. Meconium aspiration pneumonia occurs in 44%, and respiratory distress is usually evident at birth as well as meconium staining of skin, nails, and umbilical cord. The newborn will need chest physiotherapy and oxygen (usually through CPAP and sometimes mechanical ventilation). Persistent pulmonary hypertension of newborn (PPHN) may develop in response to meconium aspiration. With PPHN, the initial respiratory distress at birth often subsides and then exacerbates at 12 hours with severe respiratory distress (cyanosis, tachypnea, sternal retraction). Hypoglycemia and hypocalcemia are usually present. Treatment may include ECMO if the neonate does not respond to high-frequency ventilation.

<u>Management of Postterm Pregnancy</u>

When a pregnancy passes 42 weeks, ACOG recommends the following steps be taken:

- A woman with an unfavorable cervix may be given prostaglandin or undergo induction, or wait for spontaneous labor to start.
- The fetus should be evaluated for any signs of distress in the FHR. If distress or oligohydramnios is found, delivery should be performed.
- Fetal surveillance via a nonstress test may be performed between 41 and 42 weeks.

Prompt delivery in the event of a postterm pregnancy, favorable cervix, and no complications may be performed.

Postpartum

Postpartum Physiology

Physiological Changes

Various functions return to normal in the **postpartum period**. The thyroid level returns to normal within 4 to 6 weeks. Serum glucose levels are lower and there is a reduction in insulin requirements in diabetic women as the basal metabolic rate returns to normal during the first 7 to 14 days postpartum. Proteinuria continues for 1 or 2 days and then resolves. Diuresis begins 12 hours after birth and stops in about 5 days. Electrolytes are normal again by 21 days postpartum. Blood volume and cardiac output reaches pre-pregnancy levels by 2 to 3 weeks. Hematocrit levels drop to normal levels within 4 to 8 weeks. The respiratory system returns to normal quickly after birth with some permanent changes. The mother may find she tires quickly after exercise for the first few weeks because of respiratory changes. Tone slowly returns to the rectus muscles of the abdomen. Joint instability from pregnancy resolves by 8 weeks postpartum. Gastrointestinal tone and motility are decreased after birth and return to normal by 2 weeks.

Cervix, Vagina, Pelvic Floor, and Bladder

The cervix stays dilated until the end of the first week postpartum when it is again at 1 cm. The **vagina** may be bruised at birth. By the third week, rugae are seen again in the vaginal walls. The muscles of the **pelvic floor** regain their tone by 6 weeks postpartum. Kegel exercises can help this process. The **bladder** and **urethra** are stretched and displaced during pregnancy. Anesthesia may cause numbness soon after birth, resulting in an overdistended bladder. This should resolve within 6 to 8 hours and spontaneous voiding should resume. Traumatic effects on the **bladder** and urethra from labor gradually disappear over the first 24 hours postpartum. Bladder tone is regained within 5 to 7 days after birth.

Changes in Placental Site and Lochia

Placental separation occurs within 30 minutes of birth. The spongy layer of the endometrium of the uterus is lost at the same time, leaving decidual basalis. The top layer of the decidua dies and sloughs. The lower basal layer generates a new endometrium within 2 to 3 weeks. After separation the placental site is about 8 to 10 cm. This area shrinks to 3 to 4 cm by the end of 2 weeks postpartum. The same process occurs at the site as in the uterine walls, only more slowly. The superficial layer of the site sloughs during the first 2 weeks and new endometrium is regenerated over the next 4 weeks. During this time, tissue sloughed by the uterus is seen as **vaginal lochia**. It is reddish in color (rubra) with clots for the first 1 to 3 days after birth, then turns pink (serosa) for the next 3 to 10 days. A yellow-whitish mucus lochia (alba) will then be seen for the next 10 to 14 days or longer.

Uterine Involution

Involution begins with a decreased blood supply to the uterus. The resultant ischemia causes the release of proteolytic enzymes. These enzymes are joined by macrophages that remove tissue by phagocytosis. Some elastic and fibrous tissue remains so the uterus never goes back to its prepregnancy size. At birth the uterus weighs 1,000 g. By 24 hours after birth, it is the size it was at 20 weeks. At the end of 1 week, it is down to 500 g, and further reduces to 100 g or less at 6 weeks. The uterus can be palpated halfway between the umbilicus and symphysis pubis after birth. As the muscles relax, the fundus returns to just above the umbilical level. Uterine contractions from

- 71 -

oxytocin secretion help involution during the first few days postpartum. After the first 24 to 72 hours postpartum, the uterus begins to descend about 1 cm per day. The final size of the uterus depends on the number of pregnancies and the amount of uterine distension during the pregnancy.

Maternal Rh Alloimmunization and Indications for Rho Immune Globulin for Rh- Women

Rh incompatibility occurs if the mother is Rh- and the father is Rh+, putting their infant is at risk for hemolytic disease of the newborn (HDN) or Rh disease, (erythroblastosis fetalis). **Rh alloimmunization** (formation of antibodies against foreign antigens) can occur during abortion, abruptio placenta, amniocentesis, cesarean section, chorionic villus sampling, cordocentesis, delivery, ectopic pregnancy, and toxemia. To prevent erythroblastosis fetalis, women who are Rh- with an Rh+ mate receive the serum RhoGAM®, containing anti Rh+ antibodies. The purpose of the antibodies is to agglutinate any fetal red blood cells that pass over into the mother's circulatory system and thus prevent the mother from forming antibodies against them that will attack the infant and sensitize her for future pregnancies:

- Mother receives 300 Φg RhoGAM (RhIg, Rh immunoglobulin) intramuscularly at 26 to 28 weeks of pregnancy and again within 72 hours after her delivery.
- Miscarriage, ectopic, abortion: At ≤12 weeks, the mother receives50 Φg of MICRhoGAM®. At ≥13 weeks, the mother receives RhoGAM® as for pregnancy.

ABO incompatibility is similar but usually less severe although some infants require phototherapy for jaundice and/or exchange transfusion.

Perineal Assessment

The perineal assessment should include assessment of lochia as well as the condition of the tissue:

- **Perineum**: Perineal area should be examined and amount of swelling and bruising noted as well as condition of episiotomy (if present) and sutures. Severe perineal/rectal pain requires further examination. Rectum should be examined for presence of tearing or hemorrhoids. No severe rectal pain should be present. If hemorrhoids are present, engorgement must be reported to physician, especially if ≥2 cm in size.
- **Lochia**: Lochia should be checked every 15 minutes for signs of excess bleeding, such as copious discharge or large clots. Lochia must be observed while fundus is massaged to determine if there is free flow of blood or expulsion of clots, which may indicate hemorrhage. Lochia rubra should be present with moderate amount of discharge, <1 perineal pad/hr.

Indications for Wound Care

Wound care of the postpartum mother is needed if the woman has had a Caesarean, episiotomy, or lacerations. In all cases, the patient should receive analgesia as needed.

Wound care:

- **Caesarean**: Surgi-strips or staples may be in place and the wound covered with a sterile bandage. An ice pack may be applied 15 minutes at a time to help control pain and swelling in the first 24 hours. The initial sterile bandage is usually removed after 24 hours and then the wound left open to the air or covered with light sterile gauze. The woman is usually allowed to shower after 24 hours. The wound should be routinely checked to make sure it is intact and healing.

- **Episiotomy/Lacerations**: The suture line should be checked frequently for signs of infection, hematoma, or separation. Ice packs may be applied 15 minutes at a time for the first 24 hours to reduce swelling and pain. After 24 hours, warm Sitz baths for 20 minutes 2 to 4 times daily are usually advised, and the woman cautioned to tighten buttocks muscles when sitting down to avoid stress on suture lines.

Interventions for Postpartum Pain Control

Assess the location, intensity, frequency, and type of pain present. **Uterine pain** occurs with assessment, cramping, and massage. Slow, deep breathing and relaxation can help the mother through this pain. Be sure your hands are warm during palpation and massage to decrease comfort. Administer analgesia as ordered and teach the mother the side effects and how to take the medicine when she goes home. **Perineal pain** may be relieved by analgesics and anesthetic sprays used after pericare is performed following toileting. Ice packs are also helpful in the first 24 to 48 hours to decrease edema and inflammation. Apply moist heat via a sitz bath after the first 48 hours have passed. The accumulation of intestinal gas also causes pain in the postpartum period. The use of rocking and ambulation will help. The mother should avoid gas-producing foods until the GI tract motility resumes normal functioning.

Family Adaptation

Return of Ovulation and Need for Contraception

The resumption of ovulation and the menses are individualized in each woman. The usual time for the first menses after childbirth is 7 to 9 weeks for bottle-feeding mothers and 2 to 18 months for breastfeeding mothers. **Ovulation** may occur before the first menses but most often occurs at about 10 weeks for the bottle-feeding mother and 17 weeks for the breastfeeding mother. Since the exact time of ovulation is unknown, a woman should receive **contraceptive information** when she is released to have sexual activity or before that time if there is doubt that she will wait a full 3 to 4 weeks to resume intercourse. Breastfeeding mothers should receive progestin-only oral contraceptives. Barrier methods may also be used safely, although effectiveness is less than oral contraceptives.

Best Time for Teaching Postpartum Patients

During the immediate postpartum period the woman is focused on rest and recovery, exploration of her newborn, and acceptance and integration of the birth experience. There are also physiological changes that include temporary loss of memory and problems with attention and concentration. It is believed that higher levels of pregnenolone, allopregnanolone, and cortisol affect memory. Oxytocin also causes amnesia. Therefore, whatever is taught during the first postpartum day is not likely to be retained. Postpartum teaching should ideally begin during the **latter part of pregnancy**. Teaching in the immediate postpartum period should be accompanied by written information that the woman can review as needed at home. Family and other support persons should also receive the teaching so that they can reinforce the woman's knowledge. Postpartum visits in the home or the office are also teaching opportunities.

Symptoms Postpartum Mothers Should Report to Physician

Postpartum teaching includes a list of **symptoms** that a woman should report to her physician. They include:

- the passage of large clots, placental tissues, foul-smelling lochia, or excessive bloody discharge when the uterus is firm
- increased pain in the uterus or perineal areas
- temperature elevation to more than 100 degrees Fahrenheit
- voiding problems
- signs of shock: pallor, cool, clammy skin, increased pulse, anxiety, fainting
- signs of deep vein thrombosis: red, warm, painful areas in the calf
- signs of pulmonary embolism or amniotic fluid embolism: anxiety, dyspnea, chest pain, cough, hemoptysis, pallor

Postpartum Exercises

Kegel exercises may be done to regain pelvic muscle control. The woman should be taught to hold contraction of the muscles for at least 10 seconds and to rest at least 10 seconds between contractions. **Simple exercises** may be done during the postpartum period to increase the woman's strength and endurance. Arm raises, leg rolls, and buttock lifts may begin soon after birth. A daily walking regime is also beneficial. Abdominal exercises must wait for 4 weeks after a cesarean birth. Vigorous exercise helps the mother to resume her previous social and recreational activities and with it, her psychological well-being. Her aerobic fitness, cholesterol levels, and insulin requirements all benefit from exercise. All women should **exercise to tolerance** and stop if it causes pain or fatigue.

Family's Transition After Childbirth

The family changes in **structure** after childbirth. Roles may change if the father takes on new household duties and the mother stays at home rather than going back to work. Support from an extended family helps the new parents by reinforcing childcare traditions within the family. Stress can occur when family members place expectations on the couple. Increased contact with other new parents may change the social network of the family and old friends may be in contact less because the family's interests and priorities change to accommodate parenting demands. Financial priorities may change and cause stress as the family adapts. New parents without an extended family support network benefit from referral to new parent support groups in the community.

Postpartum Follow-up After Discharge

The new mother has problems with concentration, attention, and memory during the immediate postpartum period. Unfortunately, current postpartum stays are short and she often goes home during this time, making **postpartum teaching** difficult. Many facilities solve this problem by making **follow-up calls and visits to the home**. The AAP recommends follow-up within 48 hours of discharge when the stay was less than 48 hours after giving birth. Another important visit is made 3 to 4 days after birth, in the time when problems most often develop. Postpartum follow-up allows identification of medical problems of the mother and baby, feeding difficulties, bonding problems, caregiving inadequacies, and adaption problems within the family. Gaps in knowledge are filled by the appropriate teaching and referrals. Infant screening tests may also be completed at this time. Education about proper well-baby examinations and immunizations is also given.

Lactation

Breast Engorgement

Breast engorgement occurs when the breasts become congested with the accumulation of milk, obstruction of ducts occurs, and swelling accumulates from the blockage of lymphatic channels. It can also result from excess IV fluids given during labor. It usually occurs 2 to 3 days after birth. **Engorgement** is a normal occurrence. The areola and breast are swollen, hard, and shiny. Milk must often be hand-expressed from the area around the areola to allow the infant to latch-on. The mother should take analgesia, use ice packs, and breastfeed frequently to empty the breasts and allow the supply of milk to regulate itself.

Biospecificity of Human Milk

Human milk is designed to be uniquely nutritious to the human infant. It is easily digested because of the whey-to-casein ratio that forms soft curds in the stomach. It contains lactose as the principal carbohydrate, which supports normal gut colonization and provides galactose and glucose for brain growth. It provides the proper fatty acids for the growth of the brain, retina, and CNS of the neonate. It provides passive antibodies that the mother makes in response to the environment around herself and the neonate. Nursing forges a bond between the mother and neonate as well. The composition of breast milk changes, not just in the beginning from colostrum to transitional to mature, but even during breastfeeding and from day to day. The hind milk that comes at the end of nursing contains extra fat to help satiate the infant. Milk from preterm mothers contains higher levels of fatty acids, protein, nitrogen, lipids, immune factors, and energy to meet the needs of the premature infant.

Nutritional Needs of Lactating Women

The nutritional needs of a lactating woman include foods rich in protein, fruits, vegetables, whole grains, and dairy products. The breastfeeding woman needs about an additional 500 calories (usually 2500 to 2800 calories per day). (If obese, then additional calories may not be needed). The woman should eat 3 meals daily and two to three snacks instead of three large meals. Most foods can be eaten unless they upset the child (abdominal distention, diarrhea). Fish low in mercury should be restricted to 8 ounces per week and some fish (such as shark, sword fish, tuna steak, grouper, and Spanish mackerel) that are high in mercury should be avoided. The woman should increase fluid intake by about one quart to a total of 2.5 to 3 quarts per day. Both alcohol and caffeine can have negative effects on the newborn and should be avoided. If alcohol is drunk, breastfeeding should not be done for two hours after drinking.

Teaching Points for Women Breastfeeding for First Time

Teaching begins in the delivery room or recovery room when the nurse shows the mother how to position the infant, offer the breast, and ensure that the infant has correctly latched-on. She is then taught how to release suction with her finger and how to burp the baby between breasts. She is taught how to watch for swallowing and signs of breast milk in the baby's mouth. She is taught how long and how often to nurse. Signs of satiety and weight gain will reassure her that the infant is getting enough milk. She must be taught the appearance of colostrum, transitional, and mature breast milk. She needs to know how many wet diapers to expect and the normal color of her infant's stool. Ways to trouble-shoot problems and resources to contact for advice should be provided in written form for the new mother to take home.

Breastfeeding Techniques

During breastfeeding, the baby is turned toward the mother, with the face tilted up so they can make eye contact and the mouth slightly below the nipple, which is pointed toward the baby's upper lip or nostrils. The mother should grasp the breast using a C-hold or U-hold (to make the breast firmer) and lean toward the baby, guiding the nipple toward the infant's mouth:

- **Cradle**: The baby is cradled in the arm on the nursing side with the arm supported by a pillow. The mother uses the opposite hand to guide the nipple and positions the infant toward her.
- **Cross-cradle**: The hand on the side of the breast used is free to guide the breast while the opposite arm crosses over the baby, and the hand supports the baby's head.
- **Football**: The infant is tucked under the arm on the nursing side with the arm supporting the baby's back and the hand the head.
- **Side-lying**: The mother is reclining on her side with infant cradled by the arm on the nursing side.

LATCH Breastfeeding Charting System

LATCH is an example of a tool used to evaluate breastfeeding and to communicate the status of breastfeeding with other professionals. The tool scores the status of 5 areas involved with breastfeeding:

- **Latch**: The ability of the neonate to grasp the nipple and hold on to it and suck.
- **Audible swallowing**: Presence of spontaneous swallowing while breastfeeding.
- **Type of nipple**: Whether the maternal nipple is inverted, flat, or everted after stimulation.
- **Comfort**: The condition of the nipple and breast.
- **Hold**: Ability of the mother to hold and position the infant independently while breastfeeding.

Other tools are available and being developed. The **Preterm Infant Breastfeeding Behavior Scale (PIBBS)** is used to measure the premature infant's rooting, nipple grasp, and length of time spent sucking and swallowing.

Mastitis

Mastitis is an infection of the breast. It occurs in mothers who nurse and are primigravidas, and appears between the third and fourth weeks postpartum. Only one breast is affected usually. It is caused by *Staphylococcus aureus* that enters through cracks in the nipple. The mother will have a fever and chills. She will complain of a tender area on her breast that is red, swollen, and hard. Antibiotics are given for 7 to 10 days. Abscess formation is a complication, necessitating incision and drainage. Breastfeeding may continue if the mother and physician agree. Teach the mother how to prevent mastitis. She should wash her hands before breastfeeding, keep her breasts clean, air dry her nipples, and change her breast pads frequently. She should ensure proper latching-on of the nipple to avoid trauma and break suction with her finger when removing the infant from the breast.

Maternal Contraindications to Breastfeeding

Some maternal contraindications to breastfeeding include:

- Infection with HIV/AIDS.
- Use of antiretroviral medications.

- Active tuberculosis (not treated).
- Infection with human T-cell lymphotropic virus (II or II).
- Illicit drug use.
- Use of chemotherapeutic agents.
- Radiation therapy (may require only interruption during treatment).
- Use of other medications that pass into the breast milk and may harm the child.
- Presence of herpes on the breast.
- Presence of varicella lesions on the breast (may resume after lesions crust).

Additionally, infants with galactosemia cannot tolerate lactose, which is present in breast milk. Mothers who are ill or become pregnant while nursing should be evaluated on an individual basis to determine if they should continue to breastfeed their infants. Mothers with psychiatric disorders, such as schizophrenia or postpartum depression/psychosis, may be unable to breastfeed because of emotional disturbance as well as medications used to treat these conditions.

Care of the Non-Breastfeeding Mother

The non-breastfeeding mother should be provided the same empathy and support as breastfeeding mothers and educated about breast care. The **non-breastfeeding mother** may avoid breastfeeding because of disease, medications, death of fetus, relinquishing the child for adoption, or preference for bottle-feeding. Currently, there is no FDA-approved medication for lactation suppression, but avoiding breast stimulation and applying ice packs may help to prevent engorgement, but the woman often experiences some discomfort for about the first week. Additional education should include:

- Types of **formula** and safe preparation of concentrates and powders.
- Types of **bottles and nipples and methods of feeding**. Because formula is absorbed more slowly than breast milk, infants may experience less frequent hunger but may be at risk of dehydration if they eat less frequently than every 4 hours. The baby should be fed with the head slightly elevated. The nipple and the area above it must be filled with formula so the baby is not swallowing air. The infant should be burped after every 2 or 3 ounces of formula.

Complications

Postpartum Mood Disorders

The "**baby blues**" occur in 70% to 80% of all mothers. It is a transitory **disorder** that occurs the first few days after birth. It is a time in which her emotions are labile and alternate between joy and distress. It may be caused by the rapid decline in hormonal levels after birth. It should gradually resolve within 3 weeks after birth. Each woman should receive information about the "baby blues," and a list of resources to contact for support and help should she need it. Family members must be made aware of warning signs of depression or psychosis so that they too can alert the health care provider of persistent depression symptoms. About 30% of woman suffer a lengthy depression after childbirth and may think that it is normal if they are not informed otherwise. A small number of women suffer postpartum psychosis, which is a psychiatric emergency since the woman may harm herself or others. Hospitalization and aggressive treatment is required.

Reducing the Threat of Thrombus Formation in Pregnant and Postpartum Patients

Teach the woman who is on **bedrest** before or after childbirth to do exercises and to ambulate as allowed. Pad stirrups to prevent pressure on the popliteal areas during birth. The **postpartum woman** should not cross her legs, should not allow pressure on the backs of her knees while sitting, and should avoid extreme flexion of the legs at the hips. Support hose should be worn if the woman is at increased risk because of a previous history of thrombophlebitis. Teach the signs and symptoms of thrombophlebitis, thromboembolism, and pulmonary embolism to each woman.

Postpartal Complications

Thrombophlebitis may occur in the postpartal period with indications of septic thrombophlebitis typically evident 3 to 7 days after delivery. Clot formation occurs in the vessel walls, leading to occlusion, inflammation, and risk of **thromboembolia**. Fibrinolytic activity decreases during pregnancy to prevent hemorrhage occurring with delivery; however, this change can promote development of deep vein thrombosis and thrombophlebitis. Additionally, inactivity and bed rest increase risk. Coagulation usually returns to normal within about 3 days after delivery, so later onset often relates to other factors, such as a history of varicose veins. Superficial thrombophlebitis is usually evident by observable symptoms and poses less risk of clots breaking free and migrating than deep vein thrombosis. Indications of FVT include:

- **Femoral**: Localized pain and swelling with edema of the leg from impaired circulation, often accompanied by fever and chills.
- **Pelvic**: Abdominal pain, fever, and chills as well as generalized lethargy and malaise.

Treatment varies depending on site and type but may include heat, anticoagulation, compression (stockings), elevation of affected limb, and limitations on activities.

Endometritis

Endometritis is an infection of the uterus. It occurs more often after cesarean births than vaginal births. Fever occurs about the third day postpartum, accompanied by abdominal pain, malaise, uterine tenderness, and possibly foul-smelling lochia. Risk factors include cesarean births, prolonged rupture of membranes, protracted labor, invasive procedures during labor and delivery, excess blood loss and anemia, systemic illnesses, diabetes, kidney infections, and smoking. Historically, it has been the most common cause of maternal death after childbirth. Handwashing is the most effective way to prevent it. Many organisms cause endometritis. They reach the uterus from the lower birth canal. Antibiotics are given parenterally and the infection should respond within 48 to 72 hours.

Common Postpartal Infections

Metritis (Endometrial inflammation)	May result from C-section, PROM, repeated vaginal examination, fetal scalp electrode, instruments (forceps or vacuum), high-risk status of mother (drug use, smoker, poor nutrition), pre-existing vaginal infection, and aseptic techniques. Indications include foul or scant lochia (depending on organism), uterine tenderness, temperature elevations (sawtooth pattern) 38.3 – 40°C, tachycardia, and chills.

Parametritis (Pelvic cellulitis/ Peritonitis)	Infection of connective tissue of broad ligament or all pelvic structures may result from bacterial invasion of cervical laceration or pelvic vein thrombophlebitis. Abscess may form. Indications include chills high fever (38.9 – 40°C), abdominal pain, uterine subinvolution, local and rebound tenderness, tachycardia, abdominal distention, nausea and vomiting.
Urinary	May result from birth trauma, urinary retention, and contamination (catheter). Indications include dysuria, fever, and urinary retention.
Wound	May result from contamination of lacerations, episiotomy, and C-section incisions. Indications include erythema, local pain, purulent discharge, edema, and (rare) dehiscence.

Postpartal Bleeding Complications

Hematoma and Lacerations

A hematoma may form in the perineal area after delivery, especially if an episiotomy or **lacerations** are present. Blood oozing from lacerations may be mistaken for lochia rubra, so careful examination is needed. **Hematomas** may form anywhere from the vulva to the upper vagina because of trauma. Severe vulvar or vaginal pain that is not relieved by usual analgesia may indicate a hematoma is forming. Hematomas must be monitored carefully. Those <5 cm may resolve over time. Ice packs may help to reduce discomfort. Vital signs should be monitored carefully for signs of hemorrhage. Larger hematomas require surgical excision of the most dependent portion and drainage. The incision may be closed or left open with drains or packing to prevent recurrent hematoma. If the hematoma is at the site of the episiotomy, then the suture line must be opened to identify the site of bleeding.

Retained Placental Fragments

Retained placental fragments are the most common cause of late postpartal hemorrhage. After delivery, strong uterine contractions decrease surface area of placental attachment, causing separation, which is accompanied by bleeding and formation of a hematoma between the decidua and the placental tissue. Finally, the placental membrane peels off of the uterine wall. Signs of placental separation usually occur between 5 and 30 minutes after birth:

- Globular-shaped uterus.
- Fundus rises in the abdomen.
- Increased gush or trickling of blood.
- Umbilical cord protrudes further from the vagina.

A placenta is considered **retained** if it has not separated in over 30 minutes after delivery. Clots form about the retained segments, and when they slough away days later, excessive bleeding occurs. For this reason, careful examination of the placenta is critical. Treatment usually includes oxytocin, methylergonovine, or prostaglandins to control bleeding.

Treatment of Postpartum Hemorrhage

Postpartum hemorrhage must be dealt with quickly. It may occur within the first 24 hours postpartum or as late as 6 weeks after birth. The mother will be hypotensive with pallor and dizziness after blood loss is substantial. Treatments begin with uterotonic agents such as oxytocin, methylergonovine, or prostaglandins followed by fundal massage. A urinary catheter is inserted to keep the bladder empty. Mast trousers may be applied. Bimanual compression of the uterus, uterine packing, and surgery for ligation of blood vessels and removal of retained tissues may be done. Blood is replaced as needed along with IV fluids.

Idiopathic Cardiomyopathy of Pregnancy

Idiopathic cardiomyopathy of pregnancy develops with the last month of pregnancy or the first 5 to 6 postpartal months and is not associated with pre-existing myocarditis, endocarditis, or cardiac disease. **Idiopathic cardiomyopathy** is characterized by left ventricular systolic dysfunction. Typical symptoms are similar to heart failure and include dyspnea (the most common symptom), orthopnea, cough, palpitations, and chest pain. The heart is markedly enlarged, and the ejection fraction is less than 45%. Idiopathic cardiomyopathy increases risk of thromboembolia, so the woman is often treated with heparin. Treatment is similar to that for heart failure although if it occurs prior to delivery, ACE inhibitors are withheld because of adverse effects to the fetus. Management includes bedrest, diuretics, and digoxin. The immediate mortality rate is about 2%. In some cases, the cardiac size returns to normal, but the woman's condition still remains guarded. Sterilization is often recommended to prevent the stress of further pregnancy.

Newborn

Transition

Cardiovascular Changes in Newborn's Adaptation to Extrauterine Life

The cardiovascular system undergoes changes in the newborn's adaptation to extrauterine life. The late term fetus's right ventricle accounts for two-thirds of cardiac output and the left ventricle, one third; but after birth the output equalizes between the ventricles, and cardiac output doubles because of the extra demand for oxygen. The right ventricle predominates in the fetus and the left in the neonate. After birth, blood flow to the lungs increases, and the patent ductus arteriosus closes by about 15 hours. The fetal heart rate at the time of delivery usually varies between 110 and 160, and the newborn's heart rate is similar, 110 to 160, although the heart rate may slow to 80 when the infant sleeps and increase to 180 with crying. The strength of brachial and femoral pulses should be similar (decreased femoral pulse strength may indicate coarctation of the aorta). Heart murmurs are common within the first 24 hours, but if they persist after 48 hours, this many indicate an abnormality.

Neonatal Physiologic Adaptation

The first most critical adaptation is to clear the lungs of fetal fluid and to establish regular respirations. The umbilical vessels constrict immediately and the ductus venosus, foramen ovale, and ductus arteriosus close to establish normal neonatal circulation. The neonatal body must increase the metabolic rate, use nonshivering thermogenesis, and increase muscle activity to achieve thermoregulation. When then newborn has suffered asphyxia and is acidotic, resuscitation will be needed to establish adequate oxygenation and circulation to allow the newborn's body to make the transition to extrauterine life. When **physiological adaptation** is addressed, psychological adaptation can begin. The nurse promotes mother-baby attachment by allowing skin-to-skin contact with the mother, and allowing time for the mother and father to examine and be with the infant. Breastfeeding is promoted by encouraging the newborn to suckle as soon as the infant is stable.

Neonatal Hypoglycemia

Neonatal hypoglycemia is considered to be a blood glucose below 36 mg/dL. It occurs if there is an increased use of glucose or increased production of insulin in the neonate's body. This happens to the infant of a diabetic mother, when there are pancreatic anomalies, and from hypothermia, exchange transfusion, or malpositioned umbilical artery catheter. Asphyxia, shock, and infections can also cause the increased use of glucose. **Hypoglycemia** can also result from depleted stores or decreased production of glucose. This occurs when there has been maternal starvation or when the neonate is premature or small for gestational age. It also results from endocrine deficiency and abnormal carbohydrate or amino acid metabolism.

Newborn Assessment

Apgar Score

The Apgar score is the result of the assessment done of the neonate at 1 and 5 minutes after birth. When scores are low the assessment is repeated every 5 minutes until above 7. The **Apgar score** should not be used to indicate the need for resuscitation, nor does it give any indication of the long-term outcome for the neonate. Five areas are assessed: heart rate, respiratory rate, muscle tone, reflex irritability, and color. Each finding is scored from 0 to 2 and then the scores of all 5 areas are added together to get the Apgar score. The highest score is 10.

Common Congenital Anomalies in Newborns

Common congenital anomalies in the newborn include:

- **Neural tube defects** (such as spina bifida): May result in hydrocephalus. External sac must be protected from rupture or injury prior to surgery.
- **Cleft lip/Palate**: Special feedings techniques may be needed with cleft palate.
- **Clubfoot**: Infant may require splinting or surgical repair.
- **Hypospadias**: Severity varies, but may indicate intersex conditions if severe.
- **Congenital hip dislocation/hip d**ysplasia: Symptoms may not be evident until after the neonatal period. Suspect with breech presentation, and examine carefully.
- **Congenital heart defects**: Most common are ventricular and atrial septal defects, patent ductus arteriosis, pulmonary stenosis, tetralogy of Fallot, and transposition of the great arteries. Infants usually exhibit signs and symptoms of heart failure, especially dyspnea. Heart murmur and cardiac thrill may be present on assessment as well as tachypnea and tachycardia. Many congenital heart defects need to maintain a patent ductus arteriosus before surgical repair, but normal closure is at about 15 hours after delivery, so symptoms of congenital heart defects must be promptly identified.

Common Skin Lesions or Rashes in Newborns

Hemangioma and Café Au Lait Spots

Hemangioma is a bright red vascular tumor that occurs in 1-3% of neonates, especially in girls, preterm infants <1500 g, and those whose mothers had chorionic villus sampling. The head and neck are the most common sites. **Hemangiomas** may initially appear as a faint telangiectasia or red macule, but they proliferate rapidly during the first year after which they go through a slow involution in which they decrease in size, usually complete in 95% by adolescence.

Café au lait spots (CAL) are flat skin lesions with increased melanin content and regular or irregular borders. If the CAL spots are faint, one can use a Wood lamp to make them easier to see. Less than 3 café au lait spots have no clinical significance. However, 6 or more café au lait spots with a diameter larger than 5 mm occur in 95% of patients with neurofibromatosis type 1 (NF1), a disorder of chromosome 17.

Cutis Marmorata and Erythema Toxicum

Cutis marmorata is a disorder in which the infant's skin mottles or marbles when exposed to cold, because the superficial blood vessels dilate and contract at the same time. **Cutis marmorata** occurs in 50% of infants during the first few months of life because of immature vascular and neurological systems. In areas where vessels contract, the skin appears white or pale, and in areas where vessels dilate, the skin is pink or red. The infant's skin color returns to normal when he or she is rewarmed. **Erythema toxicum** is a skin eruption of erythematous papules, vesicles, and sometimes pustules that is essentially benign and occurs in ≥50% of newborns. It is a generalized rash that resembles that of herpes simplex, occurring on the face, limbs, and trunk (everywhere except the palms and soles of the feet). It usually occurs 2-3 days after birth. The lesions are surrounded by mottled erythematous halo of about 0.5 to 1.5 cm. Individual lesions often appear and resolve within hours but new lesions occur.

Neonatal Pustular Melanosis and Subcutaneous Fat Necrosis

Neonatal pustular melanosis is a benign rash (vesicles and macules) present at birth in about 2.2% of white infants and 4.4% of black. Usually, in preterm infants, vesicles (2-4 mm) with milky fluid are present at birth and rupture, leaving a halo of white scaly tissue and a pigmented macule at the center. Full-term infants may exhibit only the macular stage as the vesicles ruptured prior to birth. The pigmented discoloration fades with time but may persist for ≤3 months. **Subcutaneous fat necrosis** is a nodular skin lesion disorder that usually occurs ≤6 weeks of birth in full-term or post-term infants caused by necrosis of subcutaneous fatty tissue. Onset is usually between days 2-21. Subcutaneous fat necrosis is commonly associated with hypothermia, trauma to tissue from forceps, neonatal stress (various causes) and hypercalcemia. One or more lesions may develop, ranging in size from about 1 cm to many centimeters with erythema obvious over lesions. Lesions are usually rubbery and often distributed across the buttocks, upper legs, shoulders, upper back, upper extremities, and cheeks.

Gestational Age Assessment of Neonates

The AAP and the ACOG recommend that all newborns be given **gestational age assessments**. This assessment evaluates the maturity of physical and neuromuscular characteristics to determine gestational age. This determination helps to predict the neonate's risk for complications. There are tools available to use for gestational age assessments, the Dubowitz Scoring System and the New Ballard Maturational Score. The Dubowitz is best for neonates of more than 34 weeks gestation. The New Ballard Maturational Score can be used to evaluate extremely premature neonates. The best time to evaluate gestational age is between 10 and 36 hours of age for neonates more than 26 weeks gestation and within 12 hours for those who are fewer than 26 weeks.

Neonatal Thrombocytopenia

Fetal, Early Onset, and Late Onset

Causes of Thrombocytopenia in Neonates

Normal female value 150,000 to 350,000; Normal male value 235,000 to 345,000	
Fetal	Alloimmune thrombocytopenia: The mother produces antibodies specific to antigens on the neonate's platelets, which cross the placenta, causing thrombocytopenia. Autoimmune thrombocytopenia: Mothers with idiopathic thrombocytopenia purpura or lupus produce antibodies against fetal platelets. Congenital infection-mediated: CMV, rubella, and toxoplasmosis. Neonates with trisomy 18 or 21.
Early onset (<72 hours)	Placental insufficiency occurs in infants who are small for gestational age or with intrauterine growth retardation. Perinatal asphyxia. Disseminated intravascular coagulation (DIC).
Late onset (>72 hours)	Late onset sepsis. Necrotizing enterocolitis.

<u>Treatment</u>

Treatment for **thrombocytopenia** includes:

- Corticosteroids depress immune response and increase platelet count.
- Platelet transfusions: If the infant is stable, transfusion is considered when the count is less than 25,000/mcL. If the infant is unstable, a transfusion is considered when the count is less than 50,000/mcL.

Normal Range for Neonatal WBC Count

Elevation in **white blood cell** (WBC) count during early infancy is generally related to the physiological stress associated with birth and metabolic demands associated with rapid growth. Very low-birth weight infants may have decreased WBC count because the bone marrow produced more red blood cells in response to hypoxia. Normal values:

White blood cell count in newborns		
Item:	Total/Absolute	Percentage
WBCs	9100 to 30,100	n/a
Neutrophils	5.5 to 18.3	61.0%
Neutrophil Bands	0.8 to 2.7	9.1%
Neutrophil Segments	4.7 to 15.6	52.0%
Lymphocytes	2.8 to 9.3	31.0%
Monocytes	0.5 to 1.7	5.8%
Eosinophils	0.02 to 0.7	2.2%
Basophils	0.1-0.2	0.5%

Neonatal Anemia

Neonatal anemia may result from blood loss (placental abruption, placenta previa, internal hemorrhage, blood draws), increased destruction of red blood cells (hereditary blood disorders, immune hemolysis [Rh/ABO incompatibility]), or decreased production of red blood cells (anemia of prematurity, bone marrow suppression, iron deficiency anemia). Mild anemia may be asymptomatic. Symptoms with severe anemia include pallor, tachypnea, hypotension, tachycardia, apnea, metabolic acidosis, jaundice, and poor feeding. Treatment includes limiting blood draws, treating underlying cause, and partial exchange transfusions with PRBCs (for severe cases). Hematocrit below 45% at term indicates anemia.

Weeks gestation	Hemoglobin	Hematocrit	Reticulocyte count
37 to term	16.8 g/dL	53%	3-7%
32	15 g/dL	47%	3-10%
28 weeks	14.5	45%	5-10%

Neonatal Polycythemia

Polycythemia, which increases risk of hyperviscosity and blood clots, is a hematocrit greater than 65% (normal value at term is 53%). **Polycythemia** occurs in up to 5% of infants. Risk is greatest for neonates that are small for gestational age, large for gestational age, or infant of diabetic mother. Polycythemia may result from increased production of red blood cells in response to fetal hypoxia and from twin-to-twin transfusion syndrome. Polycythemia may also occur if clamping of the

- 84 -

umbilical cord is delayed. The infant may appear ruddy in appearance. Male infants may exhibit priapism. Infants may have poor feeding and may be irritable and jittery. Those with neurological involvement may have seizures or exhibit signs of a stroke (paralysis, weakness). Complications include necrotizing enterocolitis, impaired renal function, hypoglycemia, and hypocalcemia. Thrombocytopenia commonly occurs with polycythemia. The infant's vital signs and laboratory values must be monitored carefully. The current treatment for severe symptomatic polycythemia is partial exchange transfusion although there is no evidence that this affects outcome.

ABO Incompatibility

About 20-25% of pregnancies involve **ABO incompatibility**, usually with the mother type O and the fetus A or B. Anti-A and anti-B antibodies occur naturally when a woman is exposed to A and B antigens in foods or bacteria, so these antibodies can cross the placenta and result in hemolysis of fetal RBC; however, the antibodies are relatively large and do not enter the fetal circulation easily. If fetal blood leaks into maternal blood (a common occurrence), then smaller antibodies form and these can cross the placenta more easily. There is no difference in affect between the first pregnancy and subsequent pregnancies. There are rarely serious complications for the fetus although the neonate may develop hyperbilirubinemia, so the infant should be observed carefully. Only in severe cases of hemolysis (rare), does the child require exchange transfusions. Anemia may develop in the weeks after delivery because of increased rate of RBC breakdown, so the neonate should be monitored with blood counts.

Newborn Reflexes

Newborn reflexes are defined below:

- **Extrusion**: Touch tip of the tongue. The newborn should stick out the tongue.
- **Moro**: Lift the head slightly and let it fall back. The arms and legs extend and abduct, then adduct and flex.
- **Palmar grasp**: Touch the palm. The newborn will grasp the finger.
- **Rooting and sucking**: Touch the mouth or cheek. The head will turn towards the finger, open the mouth, and suck.
- **Startle**: Make a sudden loud noise. The arms and legs will abduct and flex and the newborn may cry.
- **Swallowing**: Place fluid on the back of the tongue. The newborn will swallow. Can be noted in coordination with sucking while feeding.
- **Tonic neck**: With newborn supine, turn the head to one side. The arm the head faces will extend and the opposite arm flexes.
- **Trunk incurvature**: Balance newborn prone on your hand. Stroke one side of the back. The trunk will curve towards the stroking.

Neurological Assessment of Muscle Tone

Determining the quality of muscle tone in a neonate is an important part of **neuromuscular assessment**. The child is placed supine with the head in neutral position and the nurse moves body parts (arms, legs, head) to determine if the muscle tone is flaccid, jittery, or hypertonic. Neonates are slightly hypertonic so that some resistance should be felt to movement, such as when moving a leg or straightening an arm. Tone should be symmetric. The extremities are usually flexed and legs abducted to abdomen. This assessment allows the nurse to differentiate common fine tremors or jitteriness found in neonates from seizure activity or nervous system disorders that cause muscular twitching. Normal fine tremors are usually halted by holding or flexing the extremity, while seizure activity or twitching does not resolve by holding.

Silverman-Anderson Index

The Silverman-Anderson index is a tool used to assess **neonatal respiratory status**. The upper chest is examined to see if the chest and abdomen rise together or in a see-saw pattern. The lower chest is examined for signs of intercostal retractions. The xiphoid is also examined for retractions. Nasal flaring is noted. A stethoscope is used to check for an expiratory grunt. All 5 areas are given a score from 0 to 2. A score of 0 means that there is no respiratory distress. The higher the score, the greater the respiratory distress. The Silverman-Anderson index may be repeated as needed to determine the effect of interventions on the neonatal respiratory status.

Expected Physical Findings in Preterm Infants

Physical findings in a preterm infant:

- **Skin**: Immature infants have thin, transparent skin. The vernix caseosa begins development at the beginning of the third trimester. Dried, cracked skin occurs as this protective coating disappears after the 40th week.
- **Lanugo**: Fine, usually unpigmented hairs begin to appear at 24-25 weeks of gestation and thin as the neonate matures.
- **Plantar surface of feet**: Very immature infants have no creases on the soles of their feet. Creases develop first on the anterior portion and more mature infants will have creases over the entire sole.
- **Breast buds**: Fatty tissue underneath the areola increase in size as the fetus matures.
- **Ears**: Increased cartilage content produces a more rigid pinna; ear recoil increases as the infant matures.
- **Genitalia**
  - Male: The testes descend from the abdomen into the scrotum at 30 weeks of gestation and the scrotum develops rugae as the fetus matures.
  - Female: Initially, the female fetus has a large clitoris and small labia majora. As the fetus matures, the labia majora enlarge, while the clitoris shrinks.

Complications Associated with Preterm Birth

In the United States, preterm birth (<37 weeks) is the most important factor influencing infant mortality; preterm infants account for 75-80% of all neonatal morbidity and mortality. **Complications associated with preterm birth** include:

- Respiratory distress syndrome because of inadequate surfactant production (hyaline membrane disease)
- Hypothermia because of inadequate subcutaneous fat, small amounts of brown fat, and large skin surface area to mass ratio
- Hypoglycemia secondary to poor nutritional intake, poor nutritional stores, and increased glucose consumption associated with sepsis
- Skin trauma or infection secondary to fragile, immature skin
- Periods of apnea because of an immature respiratory center in the brain
- Intraventricular hemorrhage.
- Tonic seizures.
- Birth asphyxia leading to mesenteric ischemia and risk of necrotizing enterocolitis.

- Sucking and swallowing disorders.
- Electrolyte imbalances.

The original cause of the preterm birth (such as maternal infection) may also play an integral role in the likely health problem associated with prematurity.

Feeding

Infant's Nutritional Needs

A neonate's nutritional needs must be met in order for the child to develop normally:

- **Calories**: 110 to 120 kcal /kg (50-55 kcal/lb.) per day.
- **Fluid**: 40 to 60 mL/kg (18 to 27 mL/lb.) for the first two days and then increasing to 100 to 150 mL/kg (45-68 mL/lb.) by day 7.

Breast milk is produced in three phases: **colostrum** (first 2 to 4 days) is high in immunoglobulin and provides passive immunity; **transitional milk** (3 to 14 days) has more fat, carbohydrates and colostrum; and **mature milk** (by about 2 weeks) contains about 20 kcal/oz. Formula also has about 20 kcal/oz. Initially infants nurse every 1 to 3 hours for 20 to 45 minutes taking in about 1.5 to 3 oz. each time, but then establish a more regular routine of 8 to 12 feedings in 24 hours. By two months, the infant usually takes 4 to 5 ounces with each feeding. Neonates who receive formula often take in slightly more formula with each feeding and eat less frequently (every 3 to 4 hours).

Possible Problems/Complications in Infant Feeding

Problems or complications in infant feeding may relate to problems affecting the infant, mother, or both:

- **Preterm**: Often have weak sucking and swallowing or difficulty coordinating breathing with sucking and swallowing. Feeding infants in their semi-alert state in semi-upright position reduces risk of aspiration. Limiting breast feeding to 30 minutes and/or paced feedings may help to prevent fatigue and oxygen desaturation.
- **Congenital disorders**: May need increased calories (such as with CHD), and gastroesophageal reflux is common. Some may require feeding tubes and will need to relearn sucking and swallowing.
- **Maternal**: May include sore, cracked, and bleeding nipples, breast engorgement, blocked milk ducts, and mastitis, all of which result in discomfort. Mothers must be taught about these conditions and how to treat them, as discomfort is the primary reason women stop breastfeeding. Infants may have difficulty latching on to flat or inverted nipples, and nursing with a nipple shield for the first few minutes may help elongate the nipple.

Complications

Impact of Group B Streptococcal Infection on Neonates

Group B streptococcal (**GBS**) infection was a major cause of neonatal morbidity and mortality in the past. Institution of prenatal screening and treatment has lowered the rate of GBS infection dramatically. Survival of infection with GBS can result in a neonate with intellectual disability, developmental disabilities, deafness, and blindness. Symptoms of early-onset GBS infection can occur in the first 24 hours (most common) or as late as 7 days postdelivery. Signs of pneumonia, bacteremia, or meningitis are seen. Late-onset GBS infection may occur between 1 and 12 weeks of age with the same presenting signs. Symptoms include respiratory distress, apnea, lethargy, hypotonia, pallor, hypotension, tachycardia, and temperature instability. A diagnostic evaluation is done and antibiotics are given, along with treatment for respiratory symptoms.

Hyperbilirubinemia

Hyperbilirubinemia is the presence of bilirubin in the neonate's blood that is high enough to cause jaundice of the skin. It is seen in 80% of premature infants and 60% of term infants. It is caused by physiological immaturity of the liver, short-life span of fetal red blood cells, and breastfeeding. It usually resolves in 7 to 10 days in term infants. The level is monitored to prevent kernicterus or bilirubin encephalopathy. **Pathological hyperbilirubinemia** occurs when hemolytic disease of the newborn is present, or when there are bruises or hematomas. Metabolic conditions, intestinal obstruction, infections, and respiratory distress also elevate serum bilirubin. Pathological levels rise higher than those seen with physiological hyperbilirubinemia.

Neonatal Hyperbilirubinemia

Physiologic: Hyperbilirubinemia, excess of bilirubin in the blood, is characterized by jaundice. Hyperbilirubinemia is evaluated according to the levels of direct (conjugated) bilirubin and/or indirect (unconjugated) bilirubin:

- **Direct/conjugated bilirubin levels** increase with blockage of bile ducts, hepatitis or other liver damage, including drug reaction.
- **Indirect/unconjugated bilirubin levels** increase with anemias (such as hemolytic disorders) and transfusion reactions.

Basic types of hyperbilirubinemia

Physiologic	Common in newborns and usually benign, resulting from immature hepatic function and increased RBC hemolysis. Infants have larger red blood cells with a shorter life than adults, leading to more RBC destruction and resulting in an increased load of serum bilirubin, which the liver of the newborn cannot handle. Premature infants have an even greater physiologic jaundice as their RBCs live even shorter lives than the term infant's. Onset is usually within 24-48 hours, peaking in 72 hours for full term or 5 days for preterm infants and declining within a week. Phototherapy is the indicated treatment for total serum bilirubin ≥18 mg/dL

Hemolytic, Breast-Feeding Associated, and Breast-Milk Jaundice:

Hemolytic	Caused by blood/antigen (Rh) incompatibility with onset in first 24 hours. Preventive treatment is RhoGAM® prenatally or post-natal exchange transfusion. This type of hyperbilirubinemia may also result from ABO incompatibility but rarely requires treatment other than phototherapy.
Breast-feeding associated	Relates to inadequate calories during early breastfeeding with onset on 2-3 days. This slows the excretion of stool and allows bilirubin levels to rise. More frequent feeding with caloric supplements is usually sufficient, but phototherapy may be used for bilirubin 18-20 mg/dl.

Breast milk jaundice	May result from breast milk breaking down bilirubin and its being reabsorbed in the gut. Characterized by less frequent stools and onset in 4-5th day, peaking in 10-15 days, but jaundice may persist for a number of weeks. Treatment involves discontinuing breastfeeding for 24 hours.

Indications for phototherapy and exchange transfusion: Phototherapy is commonly used to treat hyperbilirubinemia and jaundice when the total serum bilirubin (TSB) indicates the infant is at risk:

Weight = Serum bilirubin level
500 to 750 g = 5 to 8 mg/dL
751 to 1000 g = 6 to 10 mg/dL
1001 − 1250 g = 8 to 10 mg/dL
1251 − 1500 g = 10 to 12 mg dL

Phototherapy is a treatment in which the infant is placed under special lights that decrease the bilirubin levels in the blood. The infant is placed under lights with a protective mask covering the eyes to prevent retinal toxicity. The lights should be 15-20 cm above the infant. The lights convert bilirubin into a water-soluble compound that can be excreted by the liver into bile and eventually into the infant's stool. The infant is clad only in a diaper to expose the most skin to the light as possible. Exchange transfusions may be used for hyperbilirubinemia if phototherapy is ineffective. Risks associated with transfusions include vascular complications, cardiac dysrhythmias, clotting disorders, and electrolyte imbalances.

Congenital Heart Disease

Acyanotic and Cyanotic

Congenital heart disease is one of the leading causes of death in children within the first year of life. There are two main types of congenital heart disease: **acyanotic** and **cyanotic**. They may also be classified according to hemodynamics related to the blood flow pattern.

Acyanotic congenital defects	
Increased pulmonary blood flow	Atrial septal defect. Atrioventricular canal defect. Patent ductus arteriosus. Ventricular septal defect.
Obstructed ventricular blood flow	Aortic stenosis. Coarctation of aorta. Pulmonic stenosis.
Cyanotic congenital defects	
Decreased pulmonary blood flow	Tetralogy of Fallot. Tricuspid atresia.
Mixed blood flow	Hypoplastic left heart syndrome. Total anomalous pulmonary venous return. Transposition of great arteries. Truncus arteriosus. Ebstein's anomaly.

Screening Processes

The most common birth defect is **congenital heart disease (CHD)**, affecting 8 out of every thousand neonates and responsible for 30% of infant deaths each year. Screening for congenital

- 89 -

heart disease begins in the prenatal period with the ultrasound, which may show structural defects. However, some structural defects are hard to visualize, and others may be simply missed because of fetal position or gestational age. Therefore, all neonates should be screened with pulse oximetry when the neonate is 24 to 48 hours old or immediately prior to discharge. A positive finding with pulse oximetry is oxygen saturation <90%. Threshold is considered less than 95% or a difference of 4% or more between the right and left foot results. With a positive result, follow-up testing should include an echocardiogram. Testing earlier than 24 hours may miss some defects as symptoms may be delayed, so a complete physical examination of the infant is necessary, and parents/caregivers should be advised of signs and symptoms of CHD that may occur after discharge.

Respiratory Distress Syndrome, Meconium Aspiration Syndrome, and Transient Tachypnea of Newborns

Respiratory distress syndrome occurs in premature infants who do not produce enough surfactant to keep the alveoli open. The syndrome includes atelectasis, hypoxemia, hypercapnia, acidosis, pulmonary vasoconstriction, alveolar damage, and alveolar and interstitial edema. **Meconium aspiration syndrome** occurs when the fetus inhales meconium-stained fluid while in utero. The airways are obstructed, inflammation and infection occur, and respiratory distress results from pneumonitis. Lung tissue is damaged and edema enters the alveoli. The alveoli may also fill with air and rupture. **Transient tachypnea** of the newborn results when the lack of labor fails to cause lung fluid reabsorption. The neonate is born with the fluid present and has mild respiratory distress for 12 to 72 hours until all of it reabsorbs.

Respiratory Emergencies in Newborns

Birth Asphyxia

Birth asphyxia is the cause of many problems after birth. **Birth asphyxia** is defined as an event that alters the exchange of gas (oxygen and carbon dioxide). This interference with gas exchange leads to a decrease in the amount of oxygen delivered to the fetus along with an increase in the level of carbon dioxide the fetus is exposed to. This gas imbalance causes the fetus to switch from normal aerobic metabolism to anaerobic metabolism. Fetal distress results and this distress then leads to increased fetal heart rate, release of meconium into the amniotic fluid, and scalp pH <7.20. Infants experiencing birth asphyxia will often present at birth with APGAR scores that are <5 at 1 minute and <7 at 5 minutes. Symptoms include (mild) tachypnea/tachycardia; (moderate) hypothermia, hypoglycemia, respiratory distress, seizures at 12-24 hours, bradycardia; and (severe) pallor, cerebral edema, seizures, intracranial hemorrhage, and apnea. Resuscitation will vary according to the infant's condition, but warming the infant, stabilizing the glucose level, and providing oxygen or EMCO (in severe cases) may be indicated.

ALI and ARDS

Acute lung injury (ALI) comprises a syndrome of respiratory distress culminating in **acute respiratory distress syndrome** (ARDS). ARDS is damage to the vascular endothelium and an increase in the permeability of the alveolar-capillary membrane when damage to the lung results in toxic substances (gastric fluids, bacteria, chemicals, or toxins emitted by neutrophils as part of the inflammatory-mediated response) reducing surfactant and causing pulmonary edema as the alveoli fill with blood and protein-rich fluid and collapse. Atelectasis with hyperinflation and areas of normal tissue occur as the lungs "stiffen." The fluid in the alveoli becomes a medium for infection. Because there is neither adequate ventilation nor perfusion, the result is increasing hypoxemia and tachypnea as the body tries to compensate to maintain a normal paCO$_2$. Symptoms are characterized by respiratory distress within 72 hours of surgery or a serious injury to otherwise

- 90 -

normal lungs with no cardiac disorder. Untreated, the condition results in respiratory failure, multi-organ failure, and a mortality rate of 5-30%. Treatment includes surfactant replacement therapy, supplemental oxygenation/ventilation, dopamine or dobutamine, and supportive care.

Meconium Aspiration Syndrome

Meconium aspiration syndrome (**MAS**) occurs when meconium expelled in the amniotic fluid (occurring in about 20% of pregnancies) is aspirated before, during, or after birth. Blood and amniotic fluids may be aspirated as well. Some infants may present with symptoms at birth, but sometimes symptoms are delayed for a number of hours. Symptoms are similar to Transient Tachypnea of the Newborn (TTN) but more severe, and the infant appears more compromised.

Meconium Aspiration Syndrome

Symptoms	Treatments
Tachypnea with prolonged expirations. Nasal flaring and sternal retraction. Course crackles. Lethargy. Hypoxemia and hypercapnia. Cyanosis. Metabolic and respiratory acidosis (PaO_2 decreased even with 100% oxygen). Hyperventilation may occur initially with hypoventilation later. Chest x-rays may show infiltrates, atelectasis, hypoinflated areas as well as hyperinflated areas. Pulmonary hypertension. Hypothermia. Hypoglycemia. Long-term sequelae may include airway obstruction, hyperinflation, and exercise-induced bronchospasm.	Preventive suctioning of the oropharynx as soon as the head is delivered. Tracheal/bronchial suctioning to remove meconium plugs as indicated. Umbilical (arterial and venous) monitoring of ABGs. Intravenous fluids. Intubation, oxygen, assisted ventilation (CPAP at 5-7 cm H_2O), and suctioning of the trachea for infants with obstruction and respiratory distress (weak respirations, bradycardia, hypotonia). EMCO as indicated. Nitric Oxide if PPHN occurs. Antibiotic prophylaxis to prevent pneumonia. Thermoregulation. Surfactant.

Cardiovascular Emergencies in Newborns

Heart Failure

Heart failure results from the inability of the heart to adequately pump the blood the body needs. In infants, it is usually secondary to cardiac abnormalities with resultant increased blood volume and blood pressure:

- **Right-sided failure** occurs if the right ventricle cannot effectively contract to pump blood into the pulmonary artery, causing pressure to build in the right atrium and the venous circulation. This venous hypertension causes generalized edema of lower extremities, distended abdomen from ascites, hepatomegaly and jugular venous distension.
- **Left-sided failure** occurs if the left ventricle cannot effectively pump blood into the aorta and systemic circulation, increasing pressure in the left atrium and the pulmonary veins, with resultant pulmonary edema and increased pulmonary pressure. Symptoms include respiratory distress with tachypnea, grunting respirations, sternal retraction, and rales, failure to thrive and difficulty eating, often leaving the child exhausted and sweaty.

Children often have some combination of right and left-sided failure. Increased pressure in the lungs after birth may delay symptoms for 1-2 weeks.

Acute Ventricular Fibrillation or Ventricular Tachycardia

Emergency defibrillation is done to treat acute ventricular fibrillation or ventricular tachycardia in which there is no audible or palpable pulse after 1 minute of CPR. A higher voltage is generally used for defibrillation than is used for cardioversion (initial dose 2 Joules/kg), causing depolarization of myocardial cells, which can the repolarize to regain a normal sinus rhythm. Defibrillation delivers an electrical discharge usually through paddles applied to both sides of the chest. If the first shock and 1 minute of CPR are ineffective, the dose is increased to 4 Joules/kg and 1 minute of CPR, repeated if still ineffective. After 3 shocks, 1 minutes of CPR is followed with epinephrine (0.1mg/kg IV) and another minute of CPR. If still ineffective, other medications (lidocaine 1mg/kg or amiodarone 5mg/kg) may be given followed by CPR. Epinephrine may be re-administered every 3 to 5 minutes with continued CPR.

Hypotension

Hypotension is a systemic mean arterial blood pressure <2 standard deviations less that average values for gestational age. The lowest reading that is within normal limits for preterm infants is calculated as gestational age plus five. Thus, a 31-week preterm acceptable low BP would be 31-36 mm Hg. Hypotension in the neonate most often relates to dysregulation of peripheral vascular tone and/or myocardial dysfunction. **Hypotension** may also occur as the result of hypocalcemia, hypovolemic, cardiogenic, or distributive shock, so determining the cause of hypotension is critical to planning appropriate intervention. Early signs of hypotension are those of compensated shock and later signs of decompensated shock. Tachycardia, respiratory distress, pallor, lethargy, and cyanosis may be evident. Dopamine (2-20 μg/kg/min) is the most commonly used drug to treat neonatal hypotension as it improves myocardial function and improves peripheral vascular tension without causing vasodilation. Oxygen is administered to combat hypoxia as well as saline bolus (10-20 mL/kg).

Complications, Assessment, and Nursing Interventions for Infections in Newborns

Escherichia Coli (E. Coli)

Newborns who are preterm or low birth weight or whose mother experienced prolonged labor or fever are at increased risk of *Escherichia coli (E. coli)* infection. Early recognition of symptoms and alerting the physician is critical. Contact precautions must be utilized.

- **GI infection**: Symptoms include green watery, bloody diarrhea, fever, and dehydration.
- **UTI**: Symptoms, such as fever pyuria, poor feeding, and irritability, usually occurs in 2nd to 3rd week but may be earlier in preterm infants or secondary to bacteremia, so urine and blood cultures are usually done and antibiotics administered.
- **Neonatal sepsis**: Infection usually obtained intrapartum with symptoms within 6 hours of delivery: Low APGAR score, poor sucking, apnea, bradycardia, unstable temperature, vomiting, diarrhea, dyspnea. Mortality rates are higher in low-birth weight and preterm infants. Treatment is with antibiotics and supportive therapy.
- **Neonatal meningitis**: May progress from diarrhea or UTI. Onset after 48 hours usually includes neurological impairment, stupor, irritability, seizures, posturing, anterior fontanel bulging, and nuchal rigidity. Treatment is with antibiotics and supportive therapy.

<u>Varicella</u>

Chicken pox, caused by the varicella zoster virus, during the first 20 weeks of pregnancy can result in an infant with **congenital varicella syndrome**, which can cause a number of abnormalities of the skin, extremities, eyes, and central nervous system. Children are often unusually small with distinctive cicatrix scarring on the skin, and chorioretinitis. Brain abnormalities may include microcephaly, hydrocephalus, cortical atrophy, enlargement of the ventricles, and damage to the sympathetic nervous system. The child may suffer mental retardation and developmental delays as well as lack of psychomotor coordination. If the mother is infected at the end of pregnancy and develops a rash from 5 days before to 2 days after delivery, the child may develop neonatal varicella, which poses a high risk to the child with mortality rates of about 30%. Vaccination prior to pregnancy is the best preventive. Premature neonates exposed after birth with ≤28 weeks gestation or ≥28 weeks if mother has no immunity should receive varicella zoster immunoglobulin (VZIG). The nurse must provide supportive care.

<u>Hepatitis B and Common Sexually Transmitted Diseases</u>

Approximately 1% of infants have perinatal hepatitis B infections, passed to the fetus by the infected mother usually during birth (80 to 95%) although transplacental transmission is possible. The infant of an infected mother should receive hepatitis B immune globulin and hepatitis B vaccine within 12 hours of birth. Most infants with the infection are asymptomatic although some will develop chronic hepatitis and may eventually require antiviral medications and/or transplantation. If symptoms are present at birth or develop after birth they may include jaundice, abdominal tenderness, dark urine, poor feeding, and vomiting. Caregivers should be taught the signs and symptoms of hepatitis and the importance of follow-up. Most other **common sexually transmitted diseases**, such as gonorrhea and chlamydia, are spread to the neonate during delivery although syphilis is spread transplacentally. Infants should be carefully examined for evidence of eye irritation, respiratory distress, skin lesions, rash, and structural abnormalities that may indicate STDs.

Cephalohematoma and Caput Succedaneum

Caput succedaneum and cephalohematoma are both examples of head molding resulting from head trauma during birthing. They can be observed during the newborn period and appear similar on physical examination because the neonate's head is swollen:

- **Caput succedaneum** is more common. It is a collection of fluid beneath the skin, but superficial to the periosteum. It often occurs when the head presses against the dilating cervix during the birth process. Vacuum assisted deliveries also contribute to caput succedaneum. The swelling crosses suture lines. Complications are rare. Swelling usually resolves over several days.
- **Cephalohematoma** occurs when blood vessels between the skull and the periosteum rupture, causing a subperiosteal collection of blood. The swelling appears several hours after birth. It does not cross suture lines. Complications such as anemia or hypovolemia may occur if the amount of bleeding is large. The blood will eventually be resorbed and may cause jaundice secondary to break down of red blood cells.

Common Fractures in Neonates

Clavicular fracture is the most common during birth. This fracture is associated with shoulder dystocia but usually does not affect respiration. Infants are often asymptomatic but may have limited movement of arm. The infant should be evaluated for other signs of traumatic injury, given acetaminophen for pain, and the infant's arm immobilized with a figure-8 clavicle strap or by pinning the arm to clothes with the baby's shoulder elevated above heart level. The mother should be taught to carry the baby by supporting the back and shoulder. The clavicle heals in about four weeks. Breech delivery increases risk for **rib fractures**: The larger the infant, the more likely to suffer one or more fractured ribs. With multiple rib fractures, the infant will show signs of pain when moved or picked up and may develop difficulty breathing that could indicate atelectasis from the fracture. Premature infants can also develop rib fractures after birth from simple handling and chest physiotherapy due to the extremely fragile nature of these bones. Multiple fractures may indicate osteogenesis imperfecta.

Neonatal Nerve Injuries

Cranial Nerves

Injury to cranial nerves can occur during birth (the recurrent laryngeal nerve is the most common) caused by compression of the head against the sacrum during birth or from the use of forceps. Symptoms relate to the specific type of **nerve injury** but may present as temporary or permanent paralysis. Often asymmetry, drooping of eye or mouth, or failure of the eyelid to close is noted, especially when the infant cries. Traumatic injury to nerves usually **resolves** over time, beginning by the end of the first week but symptoms may persist to some degree for months. An open eye must be protected by the use of synthetic tears and patching to prevent damage. Those with injury to the laryngeal nerve may have dyspnea and dysphagia and may require small frequent feedings or enteral feedings until the condition resolves. In most cases, treatment is symptomatic with careful observation so that complications can be treated promptly.

Brachial Plexus Trauma

Trauma to the brachial plexus may cause a full-term infant to hold his/her arm adducted and internally rotated after a delivery complicated by shoulder dystocia. The **brachial plexus** is a collection of nerve tissue located in the shoulder area that is the pathway for nerves traveling from the spine to the arm and shoulder. These nerves control the movement of the shoulder and arm. Most commonly, the upper portion of this plexus is damaged, leading to weak arm muscles (Erb's palsy) with movement in the hands. The startle reflex is abnormal on the affected side, but the grasp reflex is normal. If the lower portion of the plexus is damaged, the hand is paralyzed also, and the grasp reflex is absent (Klumpke's paralysis). Most infants recover fully, but recovery depends on the degree of damage to the brachial plexus (complete tear vs. stretching). Shoulder dystocia is directly related to an infant that is large for gestational age (LGA) and experiences shoulder dislocation trying to fit through the birth canal.

NAS and Withdrawal Associated with Maternal Substance Abuse

Neonatal abstinence syndrome (NAS) includes the manifestations of withdrawal that a neonate undergoes after exposure to drugs while *in utero*. These may vary somewhat depending on the type and extent of substance abuse, which may include prescription narcotics, heroin, antidepressants, and benzodiazepines. NAS is more readily treated if the mother's substance abuse was controlled with drugs such as methadone and buprenorphine. Buprenorphine causes less severe NAS than methadone. Substance abuse may result in *in utero* growth restriction, abruptio placentae, fetal cardiac arrhythmias, preterm labor and delivery, and fetal death. Neonates often have low birth weight, small head circumference, tremors, seizures, diarrhea, and hypertonic reflexes. They may feed poorly, so they may need high-caloric formula, and may cry excessively and sleep poorly. The infant may receive drugs (morphine, methadone, and buprenorphine) to relieve withdrawal symptoms. Dehydrated infants (from diarrhea) may require IV fluids. Swaddling, kangaroo care, and maintaining a quiet dimly lit environment may help to soothe the infant.

Resuscitation

AHA/AAP/ILCOR Guidelines for Rapid Assessment of Neonate's Clinical Status

Rapid assessment (AHA/AAP/ILCOR guidelines) of a neonate's clinical status begins by determining the answer to three questions:

- Is the neonate at term gestation?
- Is there good muscle tone?
- Is the neonate breathing or crying?

If the answer to any of these if no, then the infant may require resuscitation. The infant should be dried with a towel (unless <28 gestation) and gently stimulated to trigger breathing and maintained under a heated radiant warmer or wrapped in plastic to maintain body heat. Within about 30 seconds, the infant's heart rate, respirations, skin color and muscle tone should be evaluated to determine the need for further resuscitation efforts. Note that resuscitation efforts are now the same initially whether or not the infant has been exposed to meconium, and suctioning is no longer recommended in the early resuscitation efforts as the focus is on respiratory status, as asphyxia is the primary problem encountered.

Critical Personnel for High-Risk Deliveries When Resuscitation Is Anticipated

The critical personnel that should be present at high-risk deliveries when resuscitation is anticipated will vary according to those who are available and whether or not the facility has a level III or level IV neonatal intensive care unit (NICU). Personnel may include:

- **Obstetrician**: The physician should have experience with high-risk deliveries and should prepare the mother.
- **Nurse or nurse practitioner**: Advance practice nurses with experience in neonatology should be on hand to assist with resuscitation efforts and assessment.
- **Pediatrician/Neonatologist**: A neonatologist should be present if available, otherwise, a pediatrician.
- **Pediatric specialists**: Depending on the anticipated problem, a specialist should be available. For example, if a congenital heart abnormality has been identified *in utero*, a pediatric cardiothoracic surgeon should be present to evaluate the newborn. If respiratory distress is anticipated, a pediatric pulmonologist should be present.
- **Anesthesiologist**: If immediate surgical repair may be indicated or the need for a Caesarean, an anesthesiologist may be necessary.

Minimum Neonatal Resuscitation Equipment

Minimum neonatal resuscitation equipment that should be available and assembled prior to the birth of at-risk newborns:

Temperature	Thermometer
	Warmed drying towels, warmed swaddling blankets
	Radiant warmer
	Phototherapy equipment

Respiration	Oxygen tank and hood, flow meter, humidifier, heater, tubing, nasal prongs
	Bag and mask set-up (assorted sizes)
	Laryngoscope with size 0 and 1 blades
	Endotracheal tubes, sizes 2.5—4
	Bulb syringe, suction catheters, sizes 6, 8, and 10 French, suction canister
	Cardiorespiratory monitor, oxygen analyzer
Fluids	IV needles and tubing, infusion pump, umbilical catheters (sizes 2.5 and 5 Fr)
	Blood pressure monitor, pulse oximeter
	Isotonic saline, D10W
	Sodium bicarbonate
	If transfusions are done here, blood drainage system, volume expander, and blood warmer
Drugs	Epinephrine
	Naloxone
Procedures	Various sterile surgical packs, dressings, chest tubes, scalpels, hemostat
	Arterial blood gas equipment and portable x-ray machine

Neonatal Resuscitation Process and Techniques

Neonatal resuscitation:

- Place under radiant warm to prevent cold stress and complete rapid assessment.
- HR less than 100 or absent: Apply oximeter and 3 lead ECG. Bag valve mask (BVM) at 30-60 per minute with room air.
- 30 seconds later, if HR 60 to 100, continue BVM, place an LMA, or intubate according to respiratory status. At 90 seconds, if HR less than 60, start CPR 3:1 ratio of 90 chest compressions to 30 breaths per minute if heart rate <60/min despite ventilation. Oxygen is usually administered at 100% only during CPR, then the concentration is reduced. If heart rate remains <60, epinephrine (1:10,000) at 0.01 to 0.03 mg/kg IV may be given or
- At 2 minutes, re-evaluate HR, respirations, skin color, and muscle tone. If HR <60 give 10 mL/kg IV isotonic crystalloid solution over 5 to 10 minutes or blood if blood loss is suspected.
- Assess for airway obstruction (may need suction, intubation) pneumothorax (aspirate), hypoglycemia (give 2 mL/KG bolus of D10W) and cardiac problem (give prostaglandin E).

Indications for Neonatal Transport to NICU

While protocols for neonatal transport to the neonatal intensive care unit (NICU) (level III care) may vary somewhat according to facility guidelines, usual **indications** include:

- Low birth weight <1500 g.
- Congenital defects.
- Preterm birth <32 weeks
- Respiratory distress and need for IPPV or mechanical ventilation.
- Need for exchange transfusion.
- Infectious diseases (herpes, chlamydia).
- Hypoglycemia.
- Seizures.

If no level III or level IV NICU is available in the institution where the infant is born, then the infant may require transfer by ambulance or air ambulance as soon as stabilized. Level IV facilities, often at large university hospitals, are able to provide all different pediatric specialties as well as pharmacists and nutritionists and can carry out surgical repair for congenital disease (such as heart abnormalities) or acquired conditions.

Professional Issues

Ethical principles

Beneficence and Nonmaleficence

Beneficence is an ethical principle that involves performing actions that are for the purpose of **benefitting** another person. In the care of a patient, any procedure or treatment should be done with the ultimate goal of benefitting the patient, and any actions that are not beneficial should be reconsidered. As an infant ages and/or condition changes, procedures need to be continually reevaluated to determine if they are still of benefit.

Nonmaleficence is an ethical principle that means healthcare workers should provide care in a manner that does not cause direct intentional harm to the infant/mother:

- The actual act must be good or morally neutral.
- The intent must be only for a good effect.
- A bad effect cannot serve as the means to get to a good effect.
- A good effect must have more benefit than a bad effect has harm.

Autonomy and Justice

Autonomy is the ethical principle that the individual has the right to make decisions about his/her own care. In the case of infants who cannot make **autonomous** decisions, parents or family members may serve as the legal decision maker. The nurse must keep the family fully informed so that they can exercise their autonomy in informed decision-making.

Justice is the ethical principle that relates to the distribution of the limited resources of healthcare benefits to the members of society. These resources must be distributed fairly. This issue may arise if there is only one bed left and two sick infants. Justice comes into play in deciding which infant should stay and which should be transported or otherwise cared for. The decision should be made according to what is best or most just for the infants/mothers and not colored by personal bias.

Professional/Legal Issues

Philosophy of Care in Birthing Facility

The philosophy of care in a birthing unit must be an agreement that all care given be based on evidence and national standards and guidelines. All policies and procedures should be written with the guidance of these materials. They should be reviewed as needed in the light of additional evidence and changes in guidelines by major professional organizations. These organizations include the Association of Women's Health, Obstetric and Neonatal Nurses (AWHONN), the American College of Obstetricians and Gynecologists (ACOG), the American College of Nurse Midwives (ACNM), the American Academy of Pediatrics (AAP), the American Society of Anesthesiologists (ASA), the Joint Commission (JCAHO), the Centers for Disease Control (CDC), the American Heart Association (AHA), and the Food and Drug Administration (FDA).

Medical Record Documentation

Proper documentation is a cornerstone in nursing care. It is a way to communicate patient status to other caregivers. It provides a snapshot of the patient's condition during that moment in time. It documents care given, responses to that care, and further interventions taken. **Documentation** should be as streamlined as much as possible to make efficient use of nursing time. Documentation should be thorough and provide enough information for a subsequent reviewer to reach the same conclusions as the nurse did when giving care. This is the best defense against litigation. Remember that the information you chart today may need to be reviewed by you several years from now so be sure that you document all of the information you will need to defend your actions!

Sentinel Events in Perinatal Services

A sentinel event is one that requires specific actions by a Joint Commission–accredited institution. These events are so serious that they require immediate investigation and response. The criteria for these events in perinatal services are any event that results in:

- unexpected death or loss of function
- harm due to a medication error or suicide
- maternal death during the intrapartum period
- death of a full-term infant
- infant abduction
- release of infant to the wrong family
- blood group incompatibility causing a hemolytic transfusion reaction
- wrong surgery
- retention of foreign body after surgery
- hyperbilirubinemia above 30 mg/dL

Areas of Obstetrical Nursing Most Prone to Litigation

Certain areas of care are more highly scrutinized during litigation. The policies and procedures guiding care in these areas should be reviewed continually to be sure they are in line with national standards. **Litigation** is common in the areas of FHR interpretation, documentation, and communication, telephone triage, labor induction, the use of misoprostol or oxytocin, hyperstimulation interventions, response to pain, nursing role during regional anesthesia, use of fundal pressure, interventions for shoulder dystocia, management of the second stage, use of forceps and vacuum extraction, expedited cesarean births, vaginal birth after cesarean birth (VBAC), care of multiple gestations, unintended prematurity, neonatal resuscitation, and prevention of Group B streptococcal infection in the newborn.

Evidence-Based Practice

Key Concepts

Reliability, Validity, Significance

Evidence-based practice requires the use of best evidence (based on research) in the provision of patient care. Research that is conducted or reviewed must meet standards related to:

- **Validity**: The instrument/method should accurately measure that which it is intended to measure. The evidence should clearly support the conclusions reached. Internal validity occurs if changes are the result of an independent variable and not extraneous variables. External validity occurs if results can be generalized to other subjects or settings.
- **Reliability**: An instrument/method should obtain consistent measurements over time, such as when test-retest is conducted. Validity must be considered in relation to reliability because if the instrument/method lacks validity, its reliability has little value.
- **Significance**: The importance or benefits of the study should be clearly outlined. When conducting research, the significance level refers to the alpha measurement established as meaningful prior to the beginning of the research process, usually $p = 0.05$.

Levels of Evidence

Levels of evidence are categorized according to the scientific evidence available to support the recommendations as well as existing state and federal laws. While recommendations are voluntary, they are often used as a basis for state and federal regulations:

- **Category IA** is well supported by evidence from experimental, clinical, or epidemiologic studies and is strongly recommended for implementation.
- **Category IB** has supporting evidence from some studies, has a good theoretical basis, and is strongly recommended for implementation.
- **Category IC** is required by state or federal regulations or is an industry standard
- **Category II** is supported by suggestive clinical or epidemiologic studies, has a theoretical basis, and is suggested for implementation.
- **Category III** is supported by descriptive studies (such as comparisons, correlations, and case studies) and may be useful.
- **Category IV** is obtained from expert opinion or authorities only.
- Unresolved means there is no recommendation because of a lack of consensus or evidence.

Nursing Research in Obstetrical Nursing

Nursing research provides the evidence needed to guide nursing care. It is a means by which improvements in safety of care and outcome can be achieved for obstetrical patients and their infants. It is a way to evaluate new methods, equipment, and procedures. All nurses contribute to **nursing research** when they evaluate care and outcomes and think of ways to improve these areas. They then test improvements by putting them into practice and documenting the outcomes. Evaluation points the way to a revision of the theory or evidence, and provides a basis for changes in policy and procedures.

Quality Improvement

Quality improvement is a formal method of analyzing processes and performance and taking steps to improve them in order to make them more effective, efficient, and/or cost-effective. Various methods may be utilized:

- Plan-Do-Check/Show-Act.
- Continuous Quality Improvement (CQI).
- Find, organize, clarify, uncover, start (FOCUS).
- Total quality management (TQM).
- Six Sigma and Lean Six Sigma.
- Juran's quality improvement process (QIP).

Regardless of the method chosen, the steps are similar and begin with identifying those things in need of **improvement**. This may begin with failure mode and effects analysis (FMEA), gap analysis, internal research (data analysis, surveys, interviews, observations), root-cause analysis, tracer methodology, or other methods of brainstorming. Once problems or areas for potential improvement are identified, then some method of brainstorming is used to generate solutions from which one or more is selected. Plans are formulated, tested, and implemented. Following implementation, the changes are monitored and modified as needed.

Patient Safety

Importance of Communication for Patient Safety

Many adverse incidents related to patient safety result from errors or failures in **communication**. In fact, over 30% of malpractice claims result from communication failures. Communication is especially a concern during hand-off procedures. Critical information about the patient may be undocumented, forgotten, overlooked, or misplaced. For this reason, standardized hand-off procedures, such as SBAR (Situation-Background-Assessment-Recommendation) or I-PASS (Illness severity-Patient summary-Action list-Situation awareness/Contingency planning-Synthesis by receiver) should be utilized. While an initial error in communication may not directly harm a patient, the decisions made by subsequent healthcare providers may cause harm because the healthcare providers lacked essential information. Additionally, communication failures may occur because healthcare providers don't take the time to talk with patients or family or to listen attentively and to gather their input. Problems may arise if healthcare providers fail to document medications, treatments, or observations in a timely manner. Many electronic health records utilize limited narration in favor of checklists, and checking all the boxes may become a rote activity, leading to errors.

Perinatal Patient Safety Nurse

Large birthing facilities may designate a nurse as a **perinatal patient safety nurse**. This is usually an advanced practice nurse who focuses on mother/baby safety during care. This nurse monitors nursing care for adherence to safety procedures and provides education as needed. Overall coordination of efforts to evaluate and improve care to result in a safe, optimal outcome for both mother and baby is part of this role. This complies with Joint Commission's recommendations and with the goals of Healthy People 2020 that seek to improve the nursing and medical care that is given to all persons. The unit manager and staff of smaller birthing units must take this responsibility on themselves to ensure the safety of care given in their unit.

Interprofessional Practice and Patient Safety

Interprofessional practice often begins with interprofessional education in which members of two or more professions study and learn together in order to build relationships and to have a better understanding of the contributions of each profession and the role of the profession in ensuring **patient safety**. For example, in obstetrics, an interprofessional group may include a nurse, midwife, ultrasonographer, and breastfeeding specialist. Each has a different but equally important role in patient care. A better understanding of roles and responsibilities leads to better collaboration and fewer patient safety issues. Additionally, collaboration promotes cross training and awareness of patient needs. Key elements in **interprofessional practice** include leadership (definitions, who leads and how leadership is determined), monitoring (continually assessing processes and outcomes), communication (methods and styles of effective communication), and support (mutual and organizational). Studies indicate that interprofessional education and practice especially improves communication among participants, a critical element in patient safety.

Inpatient Obstetric Nurse Practice Test

1. During labor, the relaxation technique that involves relaxing all muscles in the body except for those involved in a contraction (uterine/abdominal) is
   - a. touch relaxation
   - b. progressive relaxation
   - c. neuromuscular dissociation

2. If both parents are positive for sickle cell trait (SCT), the percentage chance that each child will develop sickle cell disease (SCD) is
   - a. 25%
   - b. 50%
   - c. 100%

3. If a fetus with electronic fetal monitoring meets the criteria for National Institute of Child Health and Human Development (NICHD) category III fetal heart rate pattern and scalp stimulation results in acceleration, this probably means that
   - a. the fetus is acidotic
   - b. the fetus is not acidotic
   - c. the acidotic status cannot be determined

4. If a preterm infant develops suspected necrotizing enterocolitis, the first intervention is to
   - a. administer antibiotics
   - b. provide electrolyte supplements with feedings
   - c. stop feeding

5. The three primary causes of thromboembolic disorders in the postpartal period are
   - a. venous stasis, hypercoagulation, and blood vessel trauma
   - b. venous stasis, uterine atony, and subinvolution
   - c. venous stasis, hypercoagulation, and subinvolution

6. If a patient has gestational diabetes but it is well controlled and without complications, induction is often carried out at
   - a. 36 weeks
   - b. 38 weeks
   - c. 40 weeks

7. Leg tremors, nausea, and vomiting are most common in the first stage of labor during the
   - a. latent phase
   - b. transition phase
   - c. active phase

8. During the birthing process, the patient frequently experiences chills during
   - a. stage 2
   - b. stage 3
   - c. stage 4

9. Miscommunication about a patient's needs is most likely to occur

    a. at times of high census
    b. at patient handoff
    c. with overworked staff

10. During the first trimester, the procedure most commonly used to confirm fetal viability is

    a. chorionic villus sampling
    b. abdominal ultrasound
    c. transvaginal ultrasound

11. The hormone primarily responsible for maintenance of pregnancy is

    a. estrogen
    b. progesterone
    c. prolactin

12. With electronic fetal monitoring, an abrupt variable deceleration often indicates

    a. cord compression
    b. fetal demise
    c. maternal hypotension

13. By day 2 after delivery, the uterus should normally descend at the rate of

    a. 0.5 cm per day
    b.1 cm per day
    c. 2 cm per day

14. A patient should be discouraged from supplementing breastfeeding with formula in the early weeks because

    a. the neonate may experience nipple confusion
    b. the neonate may develop diarrhea
    c. the neonate will have increased risk of infection

15. A newborn may require resuscitation efforts if, upon first assessment, the neonate is

    a. crying loudly
    b. silently resting
    c. posturing in a flexed position

16. Braxton-Hicks contractions may begin by week

    a. 16
    b. 20
    c. 24

17. An adverse effect of an epidural for relief of pain during labor and delivery is

    a. maternal hypertension
    b. precipitous second stage of labor
    c. bladder distention

18. Low levels of alpha-fetoprotein detected in the maternal serum screen may indicate
    a. fetal demise
    b. trisomy 21 (Down syndrome)
    c. open neural tube defect

19. Chloasma is
    a. star-shaped or branched angioma
    b. dark pigmented line from the umbilicus to the symphysis pubis
    c. dark, blotchy pigmentation of the face

20. In the nonstress test (NST), fetal heart rate acceleration without movement probably indicates
    a. adequate oxygenation
    b. fetal hypoxemia
    c. fetal metabolic acidosis

21. A pregnant patient late in the third trimester has exaggerated first and third heart sounds and a systolic murmur, probably indicating
    a. Marfan syndrome
    b. onset of heart failure
    c. normal physiological changes

22. The primary risk associated with preterm premature rupture of the membranes (PPROM) is
    a. chorioamnionitis
    b. preterm birth
    c. umbilical cord compression

23. When using vibroacoustic stimulation, the stimulator should be placed over the area of the
    a. fetal trunk
    b. uterine fundus
    c. fetal head

24. The administration of antiviral medications during pregnancy
    a. is contraindicated due to the adverse effects these drugs have on the pregnancy
    b. is proven safe and effective, as these medications are categorized as class A drugs
    c. should be within 48 hours of the onset of symptoms for maximum effect

25. The first sign of fetal hypoxia and decreasing pH is often
    a. appearance of late decelerations
    b. absent fetal breathing movements
    c. absent accelerations

26. The components of the CARE principle include communicating, advocacy, respecting, and
    a. evaluating
    b. educating
    c. enabling

27. With cordocentesis, it is most important to indicate whether the blood came from the umbilical vein or one of the arteries when testing for

    a. genetic studies
    b. fetal acid-base parameters
    c. coagulation studies

28. The complementary therapy that should be avoided during pregnancy is

    a. blue cohosh
    b. chamomile tea
    c. red raspberry herb

29. In the maternal serum screen, if the alpha-fetoprotein (AFP), human chorionic gonadotropin (hCG), and unconjugated estriol (uE3) are all decreased, this is an indication of

    a. neural tube defect
    b. trisomy 21 (Down syndrome)
    c. trisomy 18 (Edwards syndrome)

30. During a uterine contraction, the usual response of the maternal cardiovascular system is to

    a. increase blood pressure and decrease pulse
    b. decrease blood pressure and increase pulse
    c. decrease blood pressure and decrease pulse

31. When assessing the fetal heart rate pattern with electronic fetal monitoring, moderate (reassuring) variability is

    a. 1 to 5 bpm
    b. 6 to 25 bpm
    c. 15 to 40 bpm

32. If a pregnant woman smoked methamphetamine throughout pregnancy, the neonate is likely to exhibit

    a. visual disturbances
    b. intrauterine growth restriction
    c. congenital abnormalities

33. Fetal foot deformities associated with amniocentesis are more likely to occur with amniocentesis completed earlier than

    a. 14 weeks
    b. 16 weeks
    c. 18 weeks

34. If a patient had normal periods in a 28-day cycle and the last menstrual period began May 26, 2015, using Naegele's rule, her estimated date of birth is

    a. January 26, 2016
    b. March 2, 2016
    c. February 2, 2016

35. A lecithin to sphingomyelin (L/S) ratio that confirms fetal lung maturity is

    a. 1:1

    b. 2:1

    c. 3:1

36. A patient should generally plan to breastfeed her neonate

    a. 6 to 8 times a day

    b. 8 to 12 times a day

    c. 12 to 14 times a day

37. Because of changes that occur in the urinary system during pregnancy, in the postpartal period the patient is at increased risk of

    a. ureteral obstruction

    b. proteinuria

    c. over-distension of the bladder

38. In order to prevent damage to the fetus, a pregnant woman with primary or secondary syphilis should receive treatment before

    a. 16 weeks' gestation

    b. 14 weeks' gestation

    c. 10 weeks' gestation

39. The normal fetal attitude is

    a. flexion

    b. extension

    c. combination of flexion and extension

40. The uterine fundus is palpated at the umbilicus. From this assessment, the gestational age can be estimated at

    a. 12 weeks gestation

    b. 32 weeks gestation

    c. 20 weeks gestation

41. If a nonstress test (NST) is nonreactive in 20 minutes of testing, the best approach is to

    a. discontinue testing.

    b. extend the test to 40 minutes or longer

    c. retest at another time

42. Prolonged fetal hypoxia is often indicated by

    a. oligohydramnios

    b. hydramnios (polyhydramnios)

    c. amniotic fluid embolism

43. When using the fourth Leopold maneuver, the presenting part is found to be moveable, suggesting

    a. engagement

    b. nonengagement

    c. hydramnios (polyhydramnios)

44. A drug that should be avoided as a treatment for chronic hypertension during pregnancy is
   a. Labetalol
   b. Methyldopa
   c. Chlorothiazide (Diuril)

45. Proper education to post-bariatric surgery patients would emphasize that pregnancy within 18 months of surgery
   a. should be avoided due to risks imposed on both the mother and baby
   b. will require cesarean delivery, but is otherwise safe
   c. should progress normally and naturally

46. The carbon monoxide inhaled in smoking tobacco affects the fetus by
   a. stimulating release of cortisol
   b. stimulating release of epinephrine
   c. decreasing placental oxygenation

47. During a uterine contraction, the contractive force lies in the
   a. upper one-third of the uterus
   b. upper two-thirds of the uterus
   c. lower one-third of the uterus

48. Maternal alcohol intake poses special risks to the fetus because
   a. the immature system cannot metabolize alcohol
   b. the mother's nutritional status is impaired
   c. the alcohol damages the fetal liver

49. The ischial tuberosity diameter considered adequate for the diameter of the fetal head during delivery is
   a. 9.5 cm
   b. 11 cm
   c. 12.5 cm

50. The phase of the contraction cycle in which the contractions begins at the fundus and then spreads downward through the uterus is the
   a. decrement
   b. peak/acme
   c. increment

51. A common cause of fetal bradycardia is
   a. fetal head compression
   b. maternal fever
   c. maternal diabetes

52. During normal singleton pregnancy, the patient should increase caloric intake over pre-pregnant needs by
   a. 200 kcal/day
   b. 300 kcal/day
   c. 500 kcal/day

53. Nocturia in the third trimester usually indicates

    a. normal physiological changes
    b. asymptomatic cystitis
    c. pyelonephritis

54. Patients who are pregnant with twins or triplets are expected to gain

    a. 25 to 35 lb (11.3 to 15.9 kg)
    b. 35 to 45 lb (15.9 to 20.4 kg)
    c. 45 to 55 lb (20.4 to 25 kg)

55. When a patient chooses to use the Bradley method of natural childbirth, the expectation is that

    a. family and friends will gather around the bed
    b. the patient will used paced breathing
    c. the room will be dimly lit and quiet

56. The purpose of a doula is to

    a. provide physical and emotional support
    b. assist with delivery
    c. communicate for the patient

57. In a frank breech position, the fetal legs

    a. precede the buttocks into the maternal pelvis
    b. are in flexed position against the abdomen and chest
    c. extend across the abdomen toward the shoulders

58. The drug that is most commonly associated with abruptio placentae is

    a. cocaine
    b. heroin
    c. methadone

59. A patient with an incompetent cervix is especially at risk of spontaneous abortion during the

    a. first trimester
    b. second trimester
    c. third trimester

60. An early indication of maternal hemorrhage is often

    a. decreased blood pressure
    b. maternal bradycardia
    c. fetal bradycardia or tachycardia

61. The presence of fetal fibronectins in the cervicovaginal fluid between 24 and 34 weeks indicates possible

    a. preterm birth
    b. congenital defects
    c. placenta previa

62. A new mother should be advised that, by day 4 after birth, a neonate should urinate approximately

    a. 3 times daily
    b. 6 times daily
    c. 10 times daily

63. The most common initial sign of respiratory distress in a neonate is

    a. cyanosis
    b. lethargy
    c. tachypnea (more than 60 breaths per minute)

64. The two primary goals when a patient is in preterm labor are to

    a. optimize status of the fetus and prevent maternal complications
    b. delay delivery and optimize status of the fetus
    c. delay delivery and prevent maternal complications

65. The classification of placenta previa that is most likely to resolve during pregnancy is

    a. partial
    b. total
    c. marginal

66. Premature rupture of the membranes in association with high fetal station increases the risk of

    a. prolapse of the umbilical cord
    b. chorioamnionitis
    c. breech presentation

67. Following birth, damage to the neonate's upper brachial plexus (C5 to C7) is likely to result in

    a. Ipsilateral Horner syndrome
    b. Klumpke palsy
    c. Erb palsy

68. The uterine rupture classification that includes direct tearing and opening into the peritoneum is

    a. incomplete
    b. complex
    c. dehiscence

69. After birth, the first step in preventing hypothermia in a neonate is

    a. placing the infant in a radiant warmer
    b. drying and swaddling the infant
    c. placing the infant in polyethylene occlusive wrapping

70. During resuscitation of a distressed, hypoxic, bradycardic neonate, the compression-ventilation ratio should be

    a. 3:1
    b. 4:1
    c. 5:1

71. When assessing the plantar grasp reflex in a neonate, a normal response is

    a. toes remain in neutral position
    b. extension of the toes
    c. flexion of the toes

72. Asymmetry in gluteal and thigh creases in a neonate may indicate

    a. hip dysplasia
    b. spina bifida occulta
    c. cerebellar ataxia

73. A factor that predisposes a patient to uterine atony is

    a. over-distension of the uterus
    b. first pregnancy
    c. oligohydramnios

74. All HIV-exposed neonates whose mothers took antiretroviral drugs during pregnancy should receive HIV prophylaxis after delivery with

    a. both zidovudine and nevirapine
    b. nevirapine
    c. zidovudine

75. In a neonate, femoral pulses that are weaker than brachial pulses likely indicate

    a. tricuspid atresia
    b. coarctation of the aorta
    c. pulmonary stenosis

76. Bleeding that occurs after delivery when the uterus is contracted usually indicates

    a. retained placental fragments
    b. coagulopathy
    c. laceration

77. Before compressing the uterus to expel clots after delivery, it is essential to ensure that

    a. the uterus is contracted
    b. the patient has no cervical lacerations
    c. the patient receives analgesia

78. Lochia usually persists for

    a. 2 to 3 weeks
    b. 4 to 5 weeks
    c. 6 to 7 weeks

79. Diarrhea in a neonate poses a greater risk of dehydration than in older children because

    a. the intestines are relatively longer and have more surface area
    b. the intestines are relatively shorter and have less surface area
    c. the intestines are relatively the same length but less efficient

80. The A_{1c} threshold for gestational diabetes is

    a. at least 6%
    b. at least 6.5%
    c. at least 7%

81. If a patient has group B *Streptococcus* infection in the rectovaginal area at the time of birth, the neonate is at increased risk of

    a. hepatosplenomegaly
    b. chorioretinitis
    c. meningitis

82. A pregnant patient with blood pressure 150/100 mm Hg, proteinuria 0.5 g in a 24-hour specimen, normal platelet count, and normal urinary output with no complaints of pain would be classified as having

    a. hypertension
    b. mild preeclampsia
    c. severe preeclampsia

83. If a patent is receiving magnesium sulfate to prevent recurrence of seizures with eclampsia, a scheduled dose should be withheld if the urinary output is below

    a. 60 mL/h
    b. 45 mL/h
    c. 30 mL/h

84. The preexisting cardiovascular condition that places a patient most at risk during pregnancy is

    a. mitral stenosis
    b. atrial septal defect
    c. mitral valve prolapse

85. Acute Fatty Liver of Pregnancy (AFLP) is

    a. a maladaptive maternal response occurring in the early stages of pregnancy
    b. a maternal condition requiring monitoring but posing little risk to the fetus
    c. the most common cause of liver failure during pregnancy

86. Contractions that last 100 seconds with 25 seconds complete relaxation between contractions indicate

    a. normal uterine contractions
    b. hypertonic uterine contractions
    c. hypotonic uterine contractions

87. The most common irregular fetal heart rhythm is

    a. premature atrial contraction
    b. sinus bradycardia
    c. sinus tachycardia

88. When assessing fetal heart rate with a fetoscope, once the fetal heartbeat is auscultated, the next step is to

    a. count the heart rate
    b. ask the mother to hold her breath
    c. palpate the maternal radial pulse

89. Consistent late decelerations are almost always an indication of

    a. epidural anesthetic
    b. preeclampsia
    c. uteroplacental insufficiency

90. When misoprostol (Cytotec) is used for cervical ripening prior to induction with oxytocin, the oxytocin should be administered

    a. 30 to 60 minutes after last dose of misoprostol
    b. at least 4 hours after last dose of misoprostol
    c. 6 to 12 hours after last dose of misoprostol

91. During induction of labor with oxytocin, if hypertonic contractions develop, the initial response should be to

    a. reduce or discontinue oxytocin
    b. reposition the patient
    c. administer oxygen at 8 to 10 L/min

92. The subarachnoid (spinal) block is most commonly used for

    a. relief of labor pain
    b. relief of delivery pain
    c. cesarean delivery

93. Ultrasound findings that suggest that external cephalic version (ECV) may be successful include

    a. lateral fetal spine position
    b. frank breach presentation
    c. anterior placenta

94. A relative contraindication to vacuum-assisted delivery is

    a. previous attempt at delivery with forceps
    b. prolonged second stage of labor
    c. fetal compromise

95. The use of the Sellick maneuver during induction of general anesthesia for cesarean is to

    a. promote placental blood flow
    b. reduce the risk of aspiration
    c. reduce maternal respiratory depression

96. If a cesarean is carried out on a patient with an epidural in place, the patient should be told to expect

    a. addition of a subarachnoid (spinal) block
    b. mild sensations of cramping and discomfort
    c. sensations of pressure and pulling

97. Using the gravida/para/abortus (GPA) classification system, a patient classified as "gravida 5, para 3" has had

    a. 5 pregnancies and 3 deliveries at more than 20 weeks' gestation
    b. 5 pregnancies and 3 deliveries at more than 37 and less than 42 weeks' gestation
    c. 5 pregnancies and 3 live births

98. When instructing a postpartal patient about using a squeeze bottle to clean the perineum after delivery, the patient should be advised to

    a. spray the water from the back to front
    b. avoid separating the labia
    c. cleanse the perineum only after each defecation or change of peripad

99. Attachment of the mother to the neonate begins

    a. during pregnancy
    b. at birth
    c. in the postpartal period

100. In a neonate, pathological jaundice is usually evident

    a. at birth
    b. within the first 24 hours after birth
    c. within the first 24 to 48 hours after birth

101. The greatest risk of herpes simplex virus (HSV) transmission to a newborn who is delivered vaginally occurs with:

    a. an active recurrent (secondary) HSV outbreak at the time of delivery.
    b. a history of a primary HSV outbreak early in pregnancy without active disease at the time of delivery.
    c. an active primary HSV outbreak at the time of delivery.

102. The parameter of fetal heart monitoring that is most predictive of fetal compromise is:

    a. baseline fetal tachycardia.
    b. minimal or absent fetal heart rate variability.
    c. variable decelerations.

103. Women who experience precipitous labor are at increased risk for:

    a. perineal lacerations.
    b. preeclampsia.
    c. urinary retention.

104. An Rh-negative mother delivers an Rh-positive infant, and alloimmunization (production of Rh antibodies in the mother) occurs. In this case, the risk of hemolytic disease is greatest in:

    a. subsequent Rh-negative fetuses.
    b. the current Rh-positive infant.
    c. subsequent Rh-positive fetuses.

105. A patient at 34 weeks' gestation in a low-risk pregnancy who reports decreased fetal movement over the preceding hour should be instructed to:

    a. report to her primary medical provider for immediate assessment.
    b. have something to eat or drink, lie on her left side, and count fetal movements over the next 1–2 hours.
    c. increase her physical activity.

106. The nurse knows that neonatal anemia in a newborn at term is indicated by a hematocrit of less than

    a. 35%
    b. 45%
    c. 55%

107. During active labor, vomiting and irritability are most commonly observed in the obstetrical patient during the:

    a. transition phase of the first stage of labor.
    b. third stage of labor.
    c. latent phase of the first stage of labor.

108. The nurse's first response to a threatening fetal heart rate pattern on the monitor is to

    a. provide oxygen to the mother via nasal cannula and assess the fetal response
    b. assess both mother and fetus in person to rule out artifact
    c. continue to assess the monitor for five minutes to establish an accurate reading

109. The uterine contractions of true labor have which of the following characteristics?

    a. They increase in both duration and intensity as labor progresses.
    b. They decrease in intensity with rest.
    c. They are not associated with changes in the cervix.

110. The patient who delivers a fetus in a persistent face presentation can expect the newborn to have:

    a. a precipitous delivery.
    b. telangiectatic nevi ("stork bites").
    c. facial edema.

111. Reasonable suspicion that a fellow nurse is impaired as a result of alcohol dependence should be reported in which of the following circumstances?

    a. Only if the nurse's behavior places patients in imminent danger
    b. As soon as possible after the concern is identified
    c. Only if the nurse is diverting controlled substances

112. Large, flat, nonblanching, blue-gray skin lesions on the flank and buttocks region of a newborn infant are consistent with:

    a. erythema toxicum.
    b. Mongolian spots.
    c. birth trauma.

113. Domestic violence during pregnancy is associated with an increased risk of:

    a. fetal death.
    b. ABO incompatibility.
    c. post-term delivery.

114. Psychosocial assessment of the patient in active labor is:

    a. performed after the third stage of labor.
    b. an assessment of the patient's knowledge and expectations of the childbirth process.
    c. performed only in patients with a history of anxiety or depression.

115. The first stage of labor ends when the:

    a. membranes rupture.
    b. cervix is completely dilated (10 cm).
    c. infant is delivered.

116. An important initial nurse response to a nonreassuring fetal heart rate pattern is to:

    a. administer high-flow oxygen by face mask.
    b. decrease the rate of intravenous fluid administration.
    c. ensure that the patient does not change position.

117. A patient in active labor acutely develops hypotension, respiratory failure, and disseminated intravascular coagulation. This clinical picture is most consistent with:

    a. eclampsia.
    b. amniotic fluid embolism.
    c. hemolysis from Rh alloimmunization.

118. The intensity of uterine contractions can be estimated with physical assessment (during a contraction) of fundal:

    a. length.
    b. effacement.
    c. indentability.

119. A contraindication for external cephalic version of the fetus in breech presentation is:

    a. an Rh-negative patient.
    b. gestational age over 37 weeks.
    c. placenta previa.

120. The most common complication of epidural anesthesia is:

    a. maternal hypertension.
    b. fetal tachycardia.
    c. maternal hypotension.

121. The most important factor in predicting successful induction of labor is:

    a. gestational age.
    b. provider experience.
    c. cervical favorability.

122. Bright red, painless vaginal bleeding in a pregnant patient at 37 weeks' gestation should be evaluated first with:

a. ultrasound.
b. digital vaginal exam.
c. urinalysis.

123. Skin-to-skin contact between the newborn and mother helps prevent heat loss through which of the following physiological mechanisms

a. Conduction
b. Convection
c. Radiation

124. Amniotic fluid evaluation consistent with fetal lung maturity should demonstrate

a. lecithin/sphingomyelin (L/S) ratio of 1:2 and the presence of phosphatidylglycerol (PG).
b. L/S ratio of 2:1 and the presence of PG.
c. L/S ratio of 2:1 and the absence of PG.

125. During a forceps-assisted vaginal delivery, traction is applied on the forceps:

a. during contractions without the patient pushing.
b. during contractions as the patient pushes.
c. between contractions.

126. A vertical uterine incision in cesarean delivery that extends into the upper uterine segment is associated with:

a. an increased risk for uterine rupture in subsequent pregnancies compared with low transverse uterine incisions.
b. decreased blood loss compared with a low transverse uterine incision.
c. an easier repair after delivery of the infant and placenta compared with a low transverse uterine incision.

127. Immediate intervention or delivery is indicated for the ominous fetal heart rate pattern characterized by:

a. persistent early decelerations with preserved beat-to-beat variability.
b. persistent late decelerations with loss of beat-to-beat variability.
c. intermittent moderate variable decelerations with preserved beat-to-beat variability.

128. Systemic signs of illness (e.g., fever, flu-like symptoms) in the breastfeeding mother are most often associated with:

a. mastitis.
b. engorgement.
c. plugged milk duct.

129. A maneuver that is contraindicated during the management of fetal shoulder dystocia is:

a. the application of suprapubic pressure.
b. the application of fundal pressure.
c. assisting the patient into the hands and knees position.

130. Betamethasone is administered to patients with preterm labor to prevent:

a. preterm delivery.

b. chorioamnionitis.

c. neonatal respiratory distress syndrome.

131. The risk of postpartum thromboembolic complications can be reduced with:

a. postpartum bed rest

b. fluid restriction.

c. minimizing time in stirrups during vaginal delivery.

132. A patient receiving oxytocin for labor augmentation shows signs of uterine hyperstimulation with an associated nonreassuring fetal heart tracing. In this case, the nurse should do which of the following?

a. Discontinue oxytocin immediately.

b. Decrease the rate of oxytocin administration by 50%.

c. Maintain the current rate of oxytocin administration.

133. In response to fetal scalp stimulation during labor, reassuring fetal status is suggested by:

a. fetal descent, lasting 15 seconds or more.

b. decreased beat-to-beat fetal heart rate variability, with an increase of 15 beats/min or more below baseline.

c. acceleration of the fetal heart rate of 15 beats/min or more above baseline, lasting 15 seconds or more.

134. Insulin production in fetuses of women with poorly controlled diabetes mellitus in relation to infants of non-diabetic mothers is:

a. decreased.

b. increased.

c. unaffected.

135. Which of the following statements about women who have undergone cesarean delivery is correct?

a. They have a lower maternal mortality rate than with vaginal delivery.

b. They are more likely to experience incontinence in the years after childbirth.

c. They have an increased risk of placenta previa in subsequent pregnancies.

136. If a loop of umbilical cord is palpated in the vagina while the nurse is performing a cervical exam on a patient in active labor, the nurse should:

a. leave her fingers in the patient's vagina while applying pressure to the presenting fetal part.

b. assist the patient in getting into the reverse Trendelenburg position (legs lower than head).

c. apply fundal pressure to guide the presenting fetal part into the pelvis.

137. Polycythemia in the newborn infant is defined as a venous hematocrit greater than:

a. 75%.

b. 55%.

c. 65%.

138. Tocolytic medication administration for preterm labor is contraindicated in the presence of:

    a. signs of intra-amniotic infection.
    b. cervix dilated less than 4 cm.
    c. fetus weight more than 2500 grams.

139. Upright or prone maternal positioning (e.g., squat, standing, hands and knees) during active labor is often effective for managing:

    a. low amniotic fluid levels.
    b. pain associated with active labor.
    c. a precipitous delivery.

140. Discharge instructions include instructing the postpartum patient to contact her primary care provider if she develops:

    a. uterine cramps with breastfeeding.
    b. foul-smelling lochia.
    c. hemorrhoids.

141. Vaginal birth after cesarean section is most likely to be successful in the patient with:

    a. induced labor.
    b. spontaneous labor.
    c. pregnancy over 41 weeks.

142. Untreated hypothyroidism in the pregnant patient is most likely to cause abnormalities in fetal:

    a. sexual organ development.
    b. brain development.
    c. cardiac development.

143. The neonatal cardiac complication most frequently associated with maternal systemic lupus erythematosus is:

    a. heart block.
    b. ventricular septal defect.
    c. supraventricular tachycardia.

144. Induction of labor in the patient with premature rupture of membranes may be recommended to decrease the risk of:

    a. uterine atony.
    b. fetal lung immaturity.
    c. chorioamnionitis.

145. A multiple gestation pregnancy is associated with a higher incidence of:

    a. post-term delivery.
    b. placental abruption.
    c. maternal polycythemia.

146. Gestational hypertension in the pregnant patient puts the fetus at increased risk for:

    a. intrauterine growth restriction.
    b. neonatal hypertension.
    c. macrosomia.

147. Continuous fetal heart rate monitoring during labor and delivery is most appropriate for the patient who is:

    a. undergoing labor induction with intravenous oxytocin (Pitocin).
    b. pregnant for the first time (nulliparous).
    c. planning to labor in a birthing tub.

148. Early decelerations observed on fetal heart rate monitoring during labor are caused by:

    a. umbilical cord compression.
    b. uteroplacental insufficiency.
    c. fetal head compression.

149. Abrupt onset of vaginal bleeding with uterine tenderness and increased uterine tone during labor is most consistent with:

    a. placenta accreta.
    b. abruptio placentae.
    c. placenta previa.

150. A patient discharged after undergoing amniocentesis should be instructed to call the medical provider immediately if she experiences:

    a. mild cramping.
    b. fatigue.
    c. persistent clear vaginal drainage.

Answer Key and Explanations

1. C: During labor, the relaxation technique that involves relaxing all muscles in the body except for those involved in a contraction (uterine/abdominal) is neuromuscular dissociation. This method helps to relieve discomfort and anxiety and facilitates the birthing process. Progressive relaxation involves contracting and relaxing one set of muscles after another, usually beginning with the feet and moving upward. Touch relaxation involves relaxing muscles in response to a partner or coach's touch. In all cases, these techniques should be practiced as preparation for birth before labor.

2. A: If both parents are positive for sickle cell trait (SCT), the percentage chance that each child will develop sickle cell disease (SCD) is 25% while 50% will be carriers and 25% will have neither the trait nor the disease. SCD is an autosomal recessive disorder; in order to develop the disease, the child has to inherit the trait from both parents. Those who inherit the trait from only one parent are carriers but do not have the disease.

	0	SCT
0	00	0/SCT = carrier
SCT	0/SCT = carrier	SCT/SCT= SCD

3. B: If a fetus with electronic fetal monitoring meets the criteria for NICHD category III fetal heart rate pattern (which usually indicates that the fetus is acidotic) and scalp stimulation results in acceleration, this probably means that the fetus is not acidotic and that the pH has not fallen below 7.2 because accelerations are a reassuring sign. NICHD category III includes lack of variability and recurrent late or variable decelerations or bradycardia. Sinusoidal pattern is also a category III finding.

4. C: Because necrotizing enterocolitis spreads from the mucosa through the wall of the intestines, perforation and peritonitis are risks, so the first intervention is to immediately stop feeding to allow the intestines to rest, and then to provide nasogastric suction to decompress the intestines, to provide fluid resuscitation and total parenteral nutrition to prevent dehydration and malnutrition, and to provide antibiotics as indicated. If perforation occurs, then surgical intervention is indicated. Preterm infants, especially those who are formula-fed, are at increased risk of necrotizing enterocolitis.

5. A: The three primary causes of thromboembolic disorders in the postpartal period are:

- Venous stasis: Compression of vessels, prolonged standing, and inactivity or bedrest cause venous stasis, which in turn results in dilated vessels and pooling of blood, promoting thrombus formation.
- Hypercoagulation: Coagulation factors are increased while the fibrinolytic system needed to dissolve clots is depressed.
- Blood vessel trauma: Damage may occur to endothelium of blood vessels during cesarean, resulting in pelvic vein thrombosis.

6. B: If a patient has gestational diabetes but is well controlled and without complications, induction is often carried out at 38 to 39 weeks because of the increased risk of macrosomia if the pregnancy is prolonged. If there are indications for earlier delivery, then tests for fetal lung maturity should be conducted prior to induction. Many patients who required insulin during pregnancy may not require any insulin in the days after delivery because the anti-insulin factor associated with the placenta stops with placental expulsion.

7. B: Leg tremors, nausea, and vomiting are most common in the first stage of labor during the transition phase. The early first stage begins with the latent phase, during which cervical effacement and dilatation to about 3 cm occur. During the active phase, the cervix becomes completely effaced and dilates to 4 to 7 cm. During the transition phase (which some authorities fold into the active phase), the cervix completes dilation to 8 to 10 cm and birth is imminent.

8. C: During the birthing process, the patient frequently experiences chills during stage 4, which extends from the delivery of the placenta through the first 1 to 4 hours after birth. The chill that develops during this time often lasts for about 20 minutes, so care should be taken to provide the patient with a warm blanket and/or warm drinks during this period of time. The cause of the chill is not clear but may result from circulatory changes occurring after delivery.

9. B: Miscommunication about a patient's needs is most likely to occur at patient

handoff when staff members are turning over patient care to others. Information may be omitted, only partially conveyed, or misunderstood. Using a standardized format for handoff, such as the SBAR method (situation, background, assessment, recommendation/request), is one way to organize information during handoff so that critical factors are conveyed. Additionally, time should always be planned into handoff for questions and answers.

10. C: Because of the position of the uterus and gestational sac, low in the pelvis, during the first trimester, the procedure most commonly used to confirm fetal viability is the transvaginal ultrasound with viability confirmed by observing the fetal heartbeat, which should be detectable by 38 days after the last menstrual period. The transvaginal ultrasound can also help to determine the location of the pregnancy (uterine or ectopic), multiple gestations, and estimation of fetal age.

11. B: The hormone primarily responsible for maintenance of pregnancy is progesterone while estrogen is primarily responsible for growth. Estrogen and progesterone are the two primary hormones produced by the placenta during pregnancy. Progesterone increases blood flow through vasodilation. It also slows the gastrointestinal tract to ensure adequate absorption of nutrients the fetus needs to develop. Progesterone also keeps the uterine muscle relaxed to prevent the onset of labor, so progesterone levels fall when labor commences.

12. A: With electronic fetal monitoring, an abrupt variable deceleration often indicates cord compression. It may also indicate some other acute cause of sudden decreased perfusion. Abrupt decelerations usually have a V or U shape on the monitor and may or may not occur in association with uterine contractions. The onset of the deceleration to the beginning of nadir is less than 30 seconds. The deceleration is at least 15 bpm for at least 15 seconds but less than 2 minutes.

13. B: By day 2 after delivery, the uterus should normally descend at the rate of 1 cm per day. The fundus usually can no longer be palpated abdominally by about day 14, although the fundus may be slightly higher in mutiparas or with an overdistended uterus. The uterus weights approximately 1,000 g/2.2 lb immediately after delivery but returns to pre-pregnancy weight (60 g/2 oz) about 6 weeks after delivery, by which time the placental site has usually healed over as well.

14. A: A patient should be discouraged from supplementing breastfeeding with formula in the early weeks because the neonate may experience nipple confusion and have difficulty sucking because the mouth motions needed to express milk from the breast are different from those needed to control the flow of milk from an artificial nipple. (Similar problems may arise if the infant is given a pacifier.) Additionally, formula stays longer in the stomach, so the infant will get hungry less frequently, preventing the breast from receiving the stimulation it needs to produce adequate amounts of milk.

15. B: Rapid assessment (AHA/AAP/ILCOR guidelines) of a neonate's clinical status begins by determining the answer to three questions:

- Is the neonate at term gestation?
- Is there good muscle tone?
- Is the neonate breathing or crying?

If the answer to any of these if yes, then the infant may require resuscitation. The infant should be dried with a towel (unless <28 gestation) and gently stimulated to trigger breathing and maintained under a heated radiant warmer or wrapped in plastic to maintain body heat. Within about 30 seconds, the infant's heart rate, respirations, skin color and muscle tone should be evaluated to determine the need for further resuscitation efforts. Note, that resuscitation efforts are now the same initially whether or not the infant has been exposed to meconium, and suctioning is no longer recommended in the early resuscitation efforts as the focus is on respiratory status, as asphyxia is the primary problem encountered.

16. A: Braxton-Hicks contractions may begin by week 16. Estrogen causes the uterine muscles to contract, but these early contractions are irregular and usually painless until late in pregnancy, at which time the contractions may become more frequent and intense and serve to prepare the uterus for labor. Braxton-Hicks contractions usually remain irregular and last fewer than 60 seconds; however, nearing onset of labor they may be regular for short periods before decreasing.

17. C: An adverse effect of an epidural for relief of pain during labor and delivery is bladder distention. The sensation to urinate is reduced, but at the same time the mother is often receiving intravenous fluids, so the bladder should be palpated frequently and the mother assisted to urinate in order to avoid distention. Other adverse effects include maternal hypotension, usually within about 15 minutes of initiation of the epidural or intermittent bolus, but it can occur within an hour. The second stage of labor is often prolonged and the urge to push decreased because of depressed sensation.

18. B: Low levels of alpha-fetoprotein (AFP) detected in the maternal serum screen may indicate chromosomal trisomies, such as trisomy 21 (Down syndrome) or 18 (Edwards syndrome), but other findings must also be evaluated, including levels of uE3, hCG, and inhibin A. A low AFP level may also indicate gestational trophoblastic disease. In some cases, overestimation of gestational age or increased maternal weight may result in a lower than expected level in the presence of a normal fetus. Fetal demise and open neural tube defects are associated with increased AFP levels.

19. C: Chloasma (melasma gravidarum) is dark, blotchy pigmentation of the face that occurs with pregnancy, commonly referred to as the "mask of pregnancy." The pigmentation on the forehead, nose, and cheeks usually recedes after delivery, but it may recur with exposure to the sun. Vascular spiders are star-shaped or branched angiomas occurring with pregnancy. Linea nigra is a dark pigmented line from the umbilicus to the symphysis pubis, most common in pregnant patients with darker complexions.

20. A: In the nonstress test (NST), fetal heart rate acceleration without movement probably indicates adequate oxygenation. A reactive (reassuring) finding includes at least 2 fetal heart rate accelerations within a 20-minute period peaking at 15 bpm or more above baseline and persisting for at least 15 seconds. These accelerations may be accompanied with movement or without, as accelerations alone are an indication fetal health. However, if fetal movement occurs without a corresponding acceleration in heart rate, this indicates fetal hypoxemia and acidosis.

21. C: If a pregnant patient late in the third trimester has exaggerated first and third heart sounds and a systolic murmur, these findings probably indicate normal physiological changes that occur with pregnancy. As the uterus expands, it pushes against the diaphragm, forcing the heart superiorly and laterally to the left. The increased blood volume and cardiac output during pregnancy results in hypertrophy and changes in heart sounds. Most patients experience no symptoms related to these changes but some patients may experience palpitations, dyspnea, and decreased exercise tolerance.

22. B: The primary risk associated with preterm premature rupture of the membranes (PPROM) is preterm birth. PPROM is rupture of the membranes at less than 37 weeks' gestation, but risk of preterm labor is greatest if the PPROM occurs at less than 34 weeks. Both the patient and the fetus are at risk of chorioamnionitis, which may actually be the cause of premature rupture of the membranes, as well as the result. Prolonged leaking may result in umbilical cord compression and reduced lung volume, so the dangers associated with prolonging pregnancy must be balanced against complications associated with preterm birth.

23. C: When using vibroacoustic stimulation, the stimulator should be placed over the area of the fetal head. The vibroacoustic stimulation does not appear to negatively affect the fetus and may reduce testing time and nonreactive findings. Vibroacoustic stimulation is contraindicated in the presence of oligohydramnios, at less than 32 weeks' gestation, and with nonreassuring fetal heart rate or pattern. Vibroacoustic stimulation may be repeated up to 3 times at 1-minute intervals for no more than 3 seconds each time.

24. C: Antiviral medications, such as zanamivir or oseltamivir (usually preferred), are routinely administered to pregnant women who have viral infections, such as influenza or herpes. The antivirals are pregnancy class C drugs (indicating safety has not been established during pregnancy), but a number of studies seem to indicate that they do not result in adverse effects on the pregnancy (such as preterm labor or premature rupture of membranes) or on the fetus, as birth defect are within the normal expected range for mothers treated with antiviral medications. Antivirals should be administered within 48 hours of onset of symptoms (such as with influenza) if possible for maximum effect.

25. A: The first sign of fetal hypoxia and decreasing pH is often the appearance of late decelerations, which are a gradual decrease in fetal heart rate at or after the peak of a contraction with return to baseline after the contraction ends. Onset to nadir is usually more than 30 seconds and the nadir appears after the peak of the contraction. Late decelerations are usually followed by disappearance of accelerations and then absence of fetal breathing movements. Absence of fetal movement is often a late sign of acute fetal distress. When absence of fetal tone is noted, the fetus is already severely compromised.

26. C: The CARE principle is utilized to help patients take a more active role in decisions about their care. The components of the CARE principle include:

- Communicating: speaking, writing, gesturing, or other means of communicating information and understanding
- Advocacy: supporting the patient, speaking for the patient's wishes and interests, and keeping the patient informed
- Respecting: showing consideration, attention, admiration, and deference to the patient.
- Enabling/Empowering: providing information, resources, and opportunities to enable the patient to make decisions

27. B: With cordocentesis (percutaneous umbilical blood sampling [PUBS]), it is most important to indicate whether the blood came from the umbilical vein or one of the arteries when testing for fetal acid-base parameters because the umbilical arteries carry deoxygenated blood with higher levels of carbon dioxide than the umbilical vein, which carries oxygenated blood. The umbilical vein is larger and easier to access, so it is used most often for cordocentesis; with genetic studies and coagulation studies, the choice of umbilical vein or artery does not affect test outcomes.

28. A: While red raspberry herb, used to reduce nausea, and chamomile tea, used for relaxation, are essentially benign, blue cohosh, which is frequently used along with black cohosh to stimulate contractions, is not considered safe for use during pregnancy because it may be associated with maternal cardiovascular abnormalities and fetal hypoxia. Generally, patients should be advised to avoid using herbal supplements and treatments before checking with the physician or midwife.

29. C: In the maternal serum screen, if the AFP, hCG, and uE3 are all decreased, this is an indication of trisomy 18 (Edwards syndrome). Neural tube defects are indicated only by an increase in AFP; however, if other parameters are increased or decreased, this is an indication of chromosomal abnormalities. Maternal samples should be obtained between weeks 16 and 18 of gestation. A fourth marker, inhibin A, may be added to the screening test because it improves the accuracy of screening for trisomy 21, especially in patients younger than 35 years.

30. A: Because of the compression that occurs against vessels during a contraction, blood flow to the placenta slows, temporarily increasing maternal blood volume by 10% to 25%. This increase causes the blood pressure to increase during the contraction and the pulse to decrease. Because of this, assessment of a patient's vital signs should be done between contractions if possible. It is important to remember that the stress and pain associated with labor may also increase blood pressure, and blood pressure may decrease if the patient is in supine position.

31. B: When assessing the fetal heart rate pattern with electronic fetal monitoring, moderate (reassuring) variability is 6 to 25 bpm. Variability is important because it shows that the sympathetic and parasympathetic nervous systems are functioning adequately. If the fetus is hypoxic, variability decreases. A normal fetal heart rate pattern should include a baseline rate of 110 to 160 bpm, presence of variability, and presence of accelerations but no decelerations. Late decelerations are especially concerning because they last longer than the contraction.

32. B: If a pregnant woman smoked methamphetamine (a CNS stimulant) throughout pregnancy, the neonate is likely to exhibit intrauterine growth restriction (IUGR) and low birth weight. Preterm birth is also common. A small number of neonates exposed to methamphetamine exhibit withdrawal, but many women using methamphetamine also use other drugs, which may result in withdrawal. Some neonates exhibit neurobehavioral impairment, including lethargy and poor motor movement, about 48 hours after birth. The pregnant woman is also at increased risk of placental abruption.

33. A: Fetal foot deformities associated with amniocentesis are more likely to occur with amniocentesis completed earlier than 13 to 14 weeks' gestation. Incidence of hip dislocation is also increased. Amniocentesis done between weeks 15 and 16 increases risk of respiratory problems. Amniocentesis is usually done for second-trimester testing between weeks 15 and 20 because amniotic fluid volume is adequate and fetal cells are present in the fluid. Fetal amniocentesis between weeks 11 and 14 should be done only if benefits outweigh risks.

34. B: If a patient had normal periods in a 28-day cycle and the last menstrual period began May 26, 2015, using Naegele's rule, her estimated date of birth is March 2, 2016. Naegele's rule:

Begin with the day the last menstrual period started and add 7 days. Then subtract 3 months:

May 26 plus 7 days equals June 2 (6th month)

6th month – 3 months equals March 2

35. C: A lecithin to sphingomyelin (L/S) ratio that confirms fetal lung maturity is 3:1. L/S ratio is the most accurate test of fetal lung maturity and should be done if delivery is considered prior to 38 weeks' gestation. Both lecithin and sphingomyelin make up surfactants, which are necessary to keep the pulmonary alveoli open. The L/S ratio is approximately 1:1 until about week 30, at which point the lecithin level increases. A level of 2:1 usually indicates mature fetal lungs but does not confirm maturity.

36. B: A patient should generally plan to breastfeed her neonate 8 to 12 times a day. Breast milk moves through the digestive system about 2 times as fast as formula, so breastfed babies require frequent feedings, usually every 2 to 3 hours. Infants should be awakened at least every 3 hours during the first weeks of life in order to ensure adequate fluids and nutrition and stimulation of the breast in order to prevent engorgement.

37. C: Because of changes that occur in the urinary system during pregnancy, in the postpartal period, the patient is at increased risk of overdistension of the bladder. During pregnancy, the bladder increases its capacity, and the stretching results in some loss of muscle tone and sensation. After delivery, diuresis occurs rapidly with loss of fluids through the urine up to 3,000 mL per day from day 2 through day 5. Because sensation is reduced, the patient may be less aware of a distended bladder, and the urinary retention may result in urinary tract infection because of urinary stasis.

38. A: In order to prevent damage to the fetus, a pregnant woman with primary or secondary syphilis should receive treatment before 16 to 18 weeks' gestation. The fetus is rarely affected if the mother receives treatment before this time, but if the mother remains untreated, the neonate may develop congenital syphilis with a wide range of physical and mental impairments, some of which may not be evident at birth but develop in the first few months or years.

39. A: The normal fetal attitude is flexion, which allows the fetus to conform to the ovoid shape of the uterus, especially in the later months of pregnancy. Attitude is the relation of the fetal parts (head, trunk, and limbs) to each other. Usually, the fetal head is flexed toward the chest, the arms and legs flexed over the abdomen and chest, and the back is flexed in a convex C-shape at the commencement of labor.

40. C: At 20 weeks' gestation, the uterine fundus should be near the umbilicus. At 12 weeks, the fundus is at the level of the symphysis pubis and at the midpoint between the symphysis pubis and umbilicus by 16 weeks. From about week 22 to 24, the gestational age can be approximated by the number of centimeters of fundal height, so 26 centimeters usually equals 26 weeks' gestation. To measure, the tape is stretched midline up the abdomen from the superior edge of the symphysis pubis through the umbilicus.

41. B: If a nonstress test (NST) is nonreactive in 20 minutes of testing, the best approach is to extend the test to 40 minutes or longer; however, if the test remains nonreactive for an extended time, the fetus may be sleeping and the test should be rescheduled for another time or

vibroacoustic stimulation may be used to attempt to elicit fetal response. Note that if a woman is extremely obese, the thick fat pad over the abdomen may make obtaining an accurate NST difficult.

42. A: Prolonged fetal hypoxia is often indicated by oligohydramnios. Most amniotic fluid is produced by the fetal lungs and kidneys, but when hypoxia is present, the fetal circulation shifts to vital organs, such as the brain and heart, with blood flow to the lungs and kidneys restricted so that the production of amniotic fluid is curtailed or, with prolonged hypoxia, ceases. During the first trimester, the fetal skin is permeable, and amniotic fluid, derived primarily from maternal serum, diffuses in and out of the fetus. The skin is keratinized by the second trimester, and most amniotic fluid from that point derives from fetal urine.

43. B: When using the fourth Leopold maneuver, if the presenting part is found to be moveable, this suggests nonengagement. For the fourth maneuver, the examiner's hands are placed on both sides of the lower uterus and the hands moved inferiorly while palpating with the fingertips to ascertain whether the presenting part is fixed, which indicates it has passed through the pelvic inlet and is engaged, or moveable. In a primigravida, engagement usually occurs at about 37 weeks, but with subsequent pregnancies, engagement may not occur until labor commences.

44. C: A drug that should be avoided as treatment for chronic hypertension during pregnancy is chlorothiazide (Diuril) because it is associated with neonatal congenital abnormalities, as well as hypovolemia, hypoglycemia, and thrombocytopenia in the neonate. Other drugs that pose a risk of congenital abnormalities are angiotensin-converting enzyme (ACE) inhibitors and angiotensin II receptor blockers (ARBs). ACE inhibitors also increase the risk of IUGR and preterm birth. These medications should be discontinued within 2 days of confirmation of pregnancy. Beta-blockers appear to be relatively safe during pregnancy.

45. A: Patients are usually advised to avoid pregnancy for at least 18 months post-bariatric surgery to give the patient time to stabilize weight loss. Pregnancy soon after surgery may result in small-for-gestational age neonates. The primary concern with pregnancy post-bariatric surgery is the maternal nutritional status because many patients have deficiencies of protein, iron, and calcium as well as vitamin deficiencies (especially vitamins B12 and D), and their caloric intake may be 500 to 1000 kcal/day, which is not sufficient to support pregnancy. Thus, patient's nutritional status should be monitored at least every trimester. The patient may need to eat several small nutritious meals daily.

46. C: The carbon monoxide inhaled in smoking tobacco affects the fetus by decreasing placental oxygenation. Carbon monoxide binds more easily to hemoglobin than oxygen, so the oxygen-carrying capacity of the hemoglobin is reduced and less oxygen is transported to the placenta and fetus. Nicotine in tobacco stimulates the release of epinephrine, which can result in tachycardia, and causes vasoconstriction, which further impairs placental oxygenation. Nicotine also stimulates the release of cortisol, which increases blood glucose levels.

47. B: During a uterine contraction, the contractive force lies in the upper two-thirds of the uterus while the lower third of the uterus and the cervix remain passive so that the pressure from above facilitates effacement and dilatation. The myometrial cells in the upper uterus do not return to their resting state between contractions but remain shorter while the myometrial cells in the lower uterus lengthen so that some tension remains in the upper uterus to maintain and promote fetal descent.

48. A: Maternal alcohol consumption poses special risks to the fetus because the immature system cannot metabolize alcohol. Alcohol readily passes to the placenta and, because of the small fetal

size, it reaches the bloodstream faster in the fetus than the mother. The increased levels of alcohol in the blood impair development of the organs and tissues and may result in fetal alcohol syndrome (FAS), characterized by facial deformities, intellectual disability, and heart abnormalities, as well as low birth weight. The pregnancy is at risk for spontaneous abortion.

49. B: The ischial tuberosity diameter (transverse distance between the ischial tuberosities) considered adequate for the diameter of the fetal head during delivery is 11 cm. Other important measurements include the diagonal conjugate, which is the distance between the anterior surface of the sacral prominence and the anterior surface of the inferior margin of the symphysis pubis. This measure should be more than 12.5 cm. The true conjugate is the distance between the anterior surface of the sacral prominence and the posterior surface of the inferior margin of the symphysis pubis. This distance averages 10.5 to 11 cm.

50. C: There are three phases to the contraction cycle:

- Increment: The contraction begins at the fundus and then spreads downward through the uterus.
- Peak/Acme: The point at which the contraction is the strongest and most intense.
- Decrement: The uterus begins to relax as the contraction decreases in intensity.

The frequency of contractions is also noted: the duration of time from the beginning of one contraction to the beginning of the next (expressed in minutes). Duration is the length of the contraction from beginning of increment to end of decrement (expressed in seconds).

51. A: A common cause of fetal bradycardia (less than 110 bpm for at least 10 minutes) is fetal head compression; however, fetal compromise is not usually present with heart rates of 100 to 110 bpm as long as the patterns are reassuring. Other causes of bradycardia include compression of the umbilical cord, fetal hypoxia, fetal acidosis, and fetal heart block. Bradycardia may also occur during the second stage of labor when the mother is actively pushing to assist contractions as this compresses the uterine vessels.

52. B: During normal singleton pregnancy, the patient should increase caloric intake over pre-pregnant needs by 300 kcal per day. In the first two trimesters, most of the growth taking place occurs in maternal tissues; by the third trimester, the growth shifts to the fetus. The fetus takes the nutrients it needs, so much of the increased calories are to provide adequate nutrients for the mother. The increased calories should be in the form of nutritious foods (fruits, vegetables, protein sources) and simple carbohydrates should be avoided.

53. A: Nocturia usually occurs during the first and third trimesters when the patient is reclining in bed because the pressure on the pelvic vessels lessens and the blood flow to the kidneys increases. Because the glomerular filtration rate also increases in pregnancy, urine output increases, resulting in nocturia. Decreasing fluid intake in the 2 hours before bedtime and avoiding diuretic liquids (such as coffee and tea) may help alleviate the nocturia. The patient should also be advised to lean forward and backward when urinating to facilitate bladder emptying by changing the pressure of the uterus on the bladder.

54. B: Patients pregnant with twins or triplets are expected to gain 35 to 45 lb (15.9 to 20.4 kg) while a patient pregnant with a singleton should gain 25 to 35 lb (11.3 to 15.9 kg). Average weight gain for a normal singleton pregnancy during the first trimester is 2.2 to 5.5 lb (1 to 2.5 kg) and during the last two trimesters 0.9 pound (0.4 kg) per week. Women who are overweight during

pregnancy should gain only 0.66 pound (0.3 kg) per week in the last two trimesters and women who are underweight 1.1 lb (0.5 kg).

55. C: When a patient chooses to use the Bradley method of natural childbirth, the expectation is that the room will be dimly lit and quiet to promote inward relaxation with the help of a partner who coaches the patient. With this method, solitude and reducing stimuli are important so that the patient can conserve energy needed to facilitate the birthing process. Fathers/Partners are encouraged to be in the room during labor and delivery. The patient is advised to breathe normally in order to remain relaxed and ensure adequate oxygenation of the fetus.

56. A: The purpose of a doula ("woman's servant") is to provide physical and emotional support to the woman in labor and delivery. A doula is typically a friend or family member who is experienced with childbirth, but the doula has traditionally been a nonmedical person. Today, professional doulas may be trained in childbirth and different comfort techniques and establish a relationship with the patient in the last few months of pregnancy. Following delivery, they may assist the patient with breastfeeding and bonding.

57. C: Breech presentations are present in about 3% of births and more common in preterm births, fetal abnormalities, and uterine/pelvic abnormalities. Breech positions include:

- Frank: The legs are completely extended toward the shoulders and head with the buttocks presenting.
- Full/Complete: The fetus is in flexed position with the legs flexed against the abdomen and chest as in cephalic presentation except that the fetus is reversed with the head in superior position.
- Footling: One or both legs are extended and presenting through the maternal pelvis ahead of the buttocks.

58. A: The drug that is most commonly associated with abruptio placentae is cocaine, with increased risk of 10% to 19%. Cocaine is absorbed rapidly into the fetal system, and the placenta, fetus, and mother all experience the vasoconstrictive effects, with the fetus suffering from decreased oxygen saturation. The vasoconstriction may be a direct cause of the abruption as it sometimes occurs shortly after ingestion of cocaine. Cocaine is also associated with placenta previa, IUGR, precipitous delivery, and preterm labor.

59. B: A patient with an incompetent cervix, which is dilation in the absence of strong contractions, is especially at risk of spontaneous abortion during the second trimester, and patients may have a history of repeated abortions during this trimester or progressively earlier deliveries with previous pregnancies. Treatment includes placement of a pursestring suture (cerclage) at the internal os or the cervical-vaginal junction. This cerclage is usually removed at week 37 to facilitate vaginal birth but it is left in place if cesarean is anticipated.

60. C: Because of the increased maternal blood volume during pregnancy, the maternal blood pressure often remains within normal limits even with extensive blood loss, and tachycardia may occur late as well. A better early indicator is often a change in the fetal heart rate, either bradycardia or tachycardia, which suggests that the fetus is in distress because of the decreased oxygenation. Causes of maternal hemorrhage include placenta previa and abruptio placentae.

61. A: The presence of fetal fibronectins in the cervicovaginal fluid between 24 and 34 weeks indicates possible preterm birth. Fetal fibronectins are proteins that promote adherence of the fetal membranes to the uterus and are usually evident in cervicovaginal fluid up until week 20, but if

- 129 -

they are present during weeks 24 to 35, this is an indication that preterm birth may occur. If the test for fetal fibronectins is negative, then the patient is unlikely to give birth within the following week.

62. B: A new mothers should be advised that, by day 4 after birth, a neonate should urinate approximately 6 times daily. Most neonates urinate within 12 to 24 hours of birth and then urinate 1 or 2 times a day during the first 2 days; by day four, neonates should urinate approximately 6 times daily. The kidneys produce a normal urinary output of 2 to 5 mL/kg/h in a neonate. Neonates are prone to acidosis because the kidneys are less able to excrete bicarbonate than older children and adults.

63. C: While tachypnea (more than 60 breaths per minute) is common immediately after birth and during the second period of reactivity, tachypnea is also the most common initial sign of respiratory distress. Other signs of respiratory distress may include substernal and supraclavicular retractions, nares flaring (normal only during the first hour after birth), central cyanosis, grunting on expiration (commonly observed with acute respiratory distress syndrome), seesaw respirations, and asymmetric chest expansion (which may indicate a collapsed lung).

64. B: The two primary goals when a patient is in preterm labor are to delay delivery and optimize the status of the fetus. In order to delay delivery, the patient may receive a tocolytic, such as magnesium sulfate or terbutaline sulfate. To optimize fetal status, corticosteroids may be administered to promote maturation of the fetal lungs. The patient receiving a tocolytic should be placed in side-lying position to increase perfusion of the placenta and must be monitored closely.

65. C: The classification of placenta previa that is most likely to resolve during pregnancy is marginal. While it is implanted in the lower part of the uterus, it is more than 3 cm from the cervical os, so as the uterus expands with the growing fetus, the implantation moves upward, away from the cervix. A partial placenta previa has a border that is within 3 cm of the cervical os but does not completely cover it while a complete placenta previa covers the cervical os.

66. A: Premature rupture of the membranes in association with high fetal station increases the risk of prolapse of the umbilical cord because the loss of fluid causes the cord to be drawn downward past the fetus. A complete prolapse occurs when the cord appears at the vaginal opening. A partial prolapse may be felt as a pulsation corresponding to the fetal heartbeat on vaginal examination. An occult prolapse in which the cord is alongside the fetal head or shoulders is determined by fetal heart rate changes but cannot be palpated or observed.

67. C: Following birth, damage to the neonate's upper brachial plexus (C5 to C7) is likely to result in Erb palsy, which affects both the upper arm and the forearm. Movement is diminished or absent with the arm extended at the side and the forearm prone. Brachial plexus injury is associated with macrosomia, breech presentation, and shoulder dystocia. In most cases, recovery occurs within 3 to 6 months, but some infants may require surgical repair; prognosis is poor for surgical intervention. Pseudoparalysis (lack of movement because of fracture) may be misdiagnosed as brachial plexus injury.

68. B: The uterine rupture classification that includes direct tearing and opening into the peritoneum is complex rupture. Symptoms vary widely, depending on the type of rupture, but may include an internal feeling of "tearing" and increased abdominal pain. Pain may occur in the chest between the scapulae or during inspiration because of irritation of the diaphragm. If the rupture is complete, then contractions may stop, fetal heart sounds may be absent, and signs of hypovolemic shock may be evident.

69. B: After birth, the first step in preventing hypothermia (temperature less than 35°C/95°F) in a neonate is immediately drying and swaddling the infant to prevent heat loss. Polyethylene occlusive wrapping is indicated for preterm and low birth weight infants. If an infant requires resuscitation, this should be done under a radiant warmer. Normal neonatal temperature ranges from 36.5°C to 37.5°C/97.7°F to 99°F, and the environmental temperature must be maintained in that same range to maintain body temperature.

70. A: During resuscitation of a distressed, hypoxic, bradycardic neonate, the compression-ventilation ratio should be 3:1 (90 compressions to 30 breaths) with the compressions and ventilations administered sequentially to facilitate adequate ventilation of the lungs. The compression rate should be at the rate of 120 compressions per minute with ventilations of 0.5 second. Ventilation is generally begun with room air and oxygen added if oxygen saturation is inadequate. Oxygen saturation is usually monitored on the infant's right wrist or hand.

71. C: When assessing the plantar grasp reflex in a neonate, a normal response is flexion of the toes. The reflex is elicited by firmly touching the area beneath the toes. This should cause the toes to immediately flex and curl toward the bottom of the foot, similar to the palmar grasp reflex in the hand. However, if the lateral sole is stroked, this will elicit a primitive Babinski reflex in the neonate, and the toes will flare and extend while the great toe dorsiflexes.

72. A: Asymmetry in gluteal and thigh creases in a neonate may indicate developmental hip dysplasia, which is hip instability that results from the femoral head and acetabulum being misaligned. The condition worsens as the child ages. Tests to identify developmental hip dysplasia include:

Ortolani: Positive findings occur when pressure applied at the head of the femur with hips in flexed position causes posterior subluxation.

Barlow: Positive findings occur when hips are rotated through range of motion and an audible click is heard at abduction because the femoral head slips out of place.

73. A: A factor that predisposes a patient to uterine atony is anything that causes overdistension of the uterus, including multiple gestations, macrosomia, and hydramnios (polyhydramnios). The stretched myometrium is unable to contract adequately to compress vessels and prevent bleeding. Other risk factors include prolonged labor, precipitous labor, and induced or augmented labor (such as with oxytocin). Uterine atony may also result from retained placental segments. An atonic uterus may be high in the abdomen, feel soft and boggy, and fail to contract on massage.

74. C: All HIV-exposed neonates whose mothers took antiretroviral drugs during pregnancy should receive HIV prophylaxis as soon as possible after birth (within 6 to 12 hours), with zidovudine, usually for 6 weeks. A 4-week course may be given if the mother had adequate viral suppression with antiretrovirals during pregnancy. Dosage is determined by the neonate's weight and weeks of gestation at birth. If the mother was not treated with antiretroviral drugs during pregnancy, then the neonate should receive both zidovudine and nevirapine.

75. B: In a neonate, femoral pulses that are weaker than brachial pulses likely indicate coarctation of the aorta. While the patent ductus arteriosus in the neonate helps to maintain systemic circulation, when it closes, perfusion to the lower body decreases, resulting in the weaker femoral pulses. If the ductus arteriosus stays open, however, there may be right-to-left shunting with differential cyanosis with oxygenation of the lower extremities lower than to the upper. The neonate may develop indications of metabolic acidosis, heart failure, and shock.

76. C: Bleeding that occurs after delivery when the uterus is contracted usually indicates laceration, which can occur in the cervix, vagina, and perineum, and about the urethra. Bleeding is usually brighter red in color than lochia, although it may be difficult to differentiate at times. Small lacerations of the cervix with minimal bleeding are quite common and usually do not require suturing, but larger lacerations often require repair. Significant blood loss can occur if lacerations are not identified and treated.

77. A: Before compressing the uterus to expel clots after delivery, it is essential to ensure that the uterus is contracted because applying external pressure on a noncontracted uterus may result in uterine inversion. When expelling clots that may have pooled in the uterus after delivery, one hand should be placed against the uterus immediately above the symphysis pubis for support while the other hand massages and cups the fundus and gently applies steady pressure toward the lower portion of the uterus.

78. B: Lochia usually persists for 4 to 5 weeks after delivery but it may last as few as 3 weeks or as long as 6. Lochia characteristics include:

Lochia rubra (days 1 to 3): dark red with small clots. Abnormal discharge incudes large clots, bright red blood, and foul odor.

Lochia serosa (days 4 to 10): serosanguineous drainage. Abnormal discharge includes persistent red drainage, excessive drainage, and foul odor.

Lochia alba (thereafter): light yellow to white discharge in decreasing volume. Abnormal discharge includes persistent lochia serosa or return to lochia rubra, foul odor, and extended drainage.

79. A: Diarrhea in a neonate poses a greater risk of dehydration than in older children because the intestines are relatively longer and have more surface area. This increases the rate of absorption, but with diarrhea it also increases the rate of fluid loss, leading rapidly to life-threatening dehydration. Diarrhea may result in hypernatremia, so treatment includes restoration of blood volume, usually beginning with intravenous 0.9% saline and then hypotonic saline (0.3% to 0.45% in dextrose 5% in water) to slowly reduce sodium levels.

80. B: The A_{1c} threshold for gestational diabetes is at least 6.5% (usually 2 findings is diagnostic). While the A_{1c} in nonpregnant people shows the average blood glucose level over 3 months, the faster rate of red blood cell turnover during pregnancy means that the A_{1c} must be done more frequently for pregnant patients, sometimes as frequently as every week, depending on the patient's status. African Americans tend to have higher A_{1c} than non-Hispanic whites, so there is some variation according to ethnicity. Hemoglobinopathies may interfere with A_{1c} results.

81. C: If a patient has group B *Streptococcus* (GBS) infection in the rectovaginal area at the time of birth, the neonate is at increased risk of meningitis, sepsis, and pneumonia if the infection occurs within the first week, while meningitis alone is the most common with later onset. GBS infection of the mother may also result in preterm pregnancy or premature rupture of the membranes. All pregnant women should be screened for GBS infection before delivery, generally between week 35 and week 37 so that treatment can be initiated.

82. B: A pregnant patient with blood pressure 150/100 mm Hg, proteinuria 0.5 g in a 24-hour specimen, normal platelet count, and normal urinary output with no complaints of pain would be classified as having mild preeclampsia. Parameters for mild preeclampsia include blood pressure at least 140 to less than 160/at least 90 to less than 110, proteinuria at least 0.3 g to less than 2 g in 24-hour specimen (or 1+ on dipstick). Other parameters (platelets, liver enzymes, urinary output,

- 132 -

headaches, abdominal/epigastric pain, visual disturbances, pulmonary edema, heart failure, cyanosis, and fetal growth restriction) remain within normal limits or are absent with mild preeclampsia but not with severe.

83. C: If a patent is receiving magnesium sulfate to prevent recurrence of seizures with eclampsia, a scheduled dose should be withheld if the urinary output is below 30 mL/h because urinary output must be adequate for the drug to clear the system and avoid toxicity, which can result in respiratory depression. Decreased urinary output is a symptom of the disorder, not a result of treatment with magnesium. Calcium gluconate is used to treat magnesium toxicity.

84. A: The preexisting cardiovascular condition that places a patient most at risk during pregnancy is mitral stenosis. The stenotic valve lies between the left atrium and left ventricle and restricts the flow of blood from the left atrium to the left ventricle. The increased volume of blood and increased heart rate associated with pregnancy may result in pulmonary congestion and/or edema. Risk persists during labor and delivery because of the hypervolemia associated with contractions.

85. C: Acute fatty liver of pregnancy (AFLP) (the most common cause of liver failure during pregnancy) is characterized by micro-vesicular fat deposits throughout the liver that crowd out hepatocytes and interfere with liver function. AFLP, which is associated with genetic mutations, occurs in the third trimester or postpartal period. Women may exhibit nausea and vomiting, upper GI hemorrhage, coagulopathy, hypoglycemia, pancreatitis, hypoglycemia, hepatic encephalopathy (with confusion and altered mental status), hypertension, jaundice, general malaise, and renal and hepatic failure. Neonates may exhibit fatty acid oxidation defects that affect multiple body systems: cardiomyopathy, liver failure, myopathy, neuropathy, and hypoglycemia (nonketotic). Some may die *in utero* and 15% after birth.

86. B: Contractions that last 100 seconds with 25 seconds complete relaxation between contractions indicate hypertonic uterine contractions because they last longer than 90 seconds and relaxation time is less than 30 seconds. The fetus has enough oxygen reserve for 1 to 2 minutes during contractions, but if the uterus does not adequately relax during between contractions, there may be insufficient time for reoxygenation, and the fetus may show signs of distress, especially if reserves are on the low side.

87. A: The most common irregular fetal heart rhythm is the premature atrial contraction (PAC). PACs often resolve without intervention, especially if they are isolated; however, PACs increase the risk of tachyarrhythmia and may be associated with cardiac abnormalities, so they should be assessed by fetal echocardiogram. Patients whose fetuses exhibit PACs are advised to avoid caffeine and drugs that are stimulant compounds, such as beta-adrenoceptor agonists, and should be advised to note indications of tachyarrhythmias, such as increased fetal activity and increased abdominal diameter from hydramnios.

88. C: When assessing fetal heart rate with a fetoscope, once the fetal heartbeat is auscultated, the next step is to palpate the maternal radial pulse to ensure that the heartbeat that is heard is actually that of the fetus and not the mother. If the mother's heart rate corresponds exactly with the heart rate heard through the fetoscope, then the fetoscope should be moved to another position until the actual fetal heartbeat is obtained.

89. C: Consistent late decelerations are almost always an indication of uteroplacental insufficiency of some kind, indicating that the fetus is not adequately oxygenated. While the late deceleration is similar in appearance to an early deceleration, it begins after the uterine contraction starts and the nadir is after the contraction stops. If an occasional late deceleration occurs with variability, it is

usually not cause for concern, but a consistent pattern with little or no variability and without accelerations requires immediate intervention.

90. B: When misoprostol (Cytotec), a prostaglandin E1 analogue, is used for cervical ripening at or near term prior to induction with oxytocin, the oxytocin should be administered at least 4 hours after last dose of misoprostol. If a dinoprostone insert (Cervidil) is used for cervical ripening, then oxytocin is administered 30 to 60 minutes after the insert is removed. With dinoprostone gel (Prepidil), oxytocin is generally administered after a 6- to 12-hour waiting period.

91. A: During induction of labor with oxytocin, if hypertonic contractions develop, the initial response should be to immediately reduce the dosage of or discontinue oxytocin. Then, the primary intravenous solution should be increased and the patient repositioned into a side-lying position to reduce pressure on the vena cava and aorta. In order to promote maternal oxygenation and oxygenation of the fetus, the patient should be administered oxygen at 8 to 10 L/min.

92. C: The subarachnoid (spinal) block is most commonly used for cesarean delivery; it generally has been replaced by the epidural for other uses because the epidural relieves pain during labor and delivery, while the subarachnoid block is administered immediately prior to delivery. The subarachnoid block results in loss of both motor and sensory function inferior to the block. Adverse effects include maternal hypotension, bladder distention, and postspinal headache because of leakage of cerebrospinal fluid at the injection site.

93. A: Ultrasound findings that suggest that external cephalic version (ECV) may be successful include lateral fetal spine position because the physician/midwife can more readily flex the fetal head, facilitating movement because the fetus is more compact. Other factors include an amniotic fluid index of more than 10 cm and posterior implantation of the placenta. Of the four breech positions, the complete breech presentation is the easiest to reposition. Maternal factors that facilitate ECV include weight 75 kg or less, multiparity, noncontracted uterus, nonengagement, and fetus positioned so head is palpable.

94. A: Because greater force can usually be applied for extraction of a fetus with forceps-assisted delivery, if this procedure fails, then use of vacuum-assisted delivery is generally contraindicated, and delivery should be completed by cesarean. Vacuum-assisted delivery is usually done for a prolonged second stage of labor that is not progressing adequately or when fetal compromise indicates the need for rapid delivery. Vacuum-assisted delivery is contraindicated with cephalopelvic disproportion, macrosomia, and inappropriate presentation.

95. B: The use of the Sellick maneuver, which involves using cricoid pressure against the trachea to effectively block the esophagus, during induction of general anesthesia for cesarean is to reduce the risk of aspiration. General anesthesia is often done in emergent situations, such as fetal compromise, and the patient may not have been NPO (nothing by mouth); so drugs may also be administered to increase the gastric pH (sodium citrate), to decrease secretions (glycopyrrolate), and to speed gastric emptying (metoclopramide).

96. C: While epidural anesthesia is adequate for cesarean, the patient should be reassured and told to expect some feeling of pressure and pulling. The patient should not experience pain during the procedure and, in some cases, may opt to watch the delivery. The nurse should remain with the patient during preparation for the operative delivery and should answer all questions and provide information about the procedures to help allay the patient and her partner's fears.

97. A: "Gravida" (G) refers to the number of pregnancies while "para" (P) refers to the number of deliveries at more than 20 weeks' gestation but does not indicate if the deliveries were full-term or

live births. Gravida and para are part of the GPA system that includes abortus as the third parameter, although this term is often omitted with live births. For example, if the patient had 5 pregnancies, 3 deliveries at more than 20 weeks, and 2 miscarriages/abortions, the classification would be G5, P3, A2.

98. B: When instructing a postpartal patient about using a squeeze bottle to clean the perineum after delivery, the patient should be advised to avoid separating the labia so that contaminated water isn't sprayed into the vagina, increasing the risk of infection. The patient should be advised to always spray the water and wipe dry from front to back to avoid fecal contamination of the vagina. The perineum should be cleaned after each urination and each defecation, and the peripad should be changed each time as well.

99. A: Attachment of the mother to the neonate begins during pregnancy when the mother makes plans for the infant and creates a fantasy image of the infant and the life they will have. Attachment is a progressive activity that is reciprocal and develops over time. Bonding, which is the initial attraction the mother feels for the infant, is enhanced if the mother and infant are allowed to interact through touch and eye contact during the first 30 to 60 minutes after birth. Bonding facilitates attachment.

100. B: Pathological jaundice is usually evident within the first 24 hours after birth while physiological jaundice, which occurs in up to 80% of neonates, is evident between 24 and 48 hours after birth. Pathological jaundice may result in rapid increase of total serum bilirubin; it is diagnosed at peak bilirubin levels more than 12.9 mg/dL in a full-term infant and more than 15 mg/dL in a preterm infant. Conditions that result in accelerated breakdown of red blood cells, such as polycythemia, birth trauma, and Rh incompatibility increase bilirubin levels.

101. C: The greatest risk to the newborn infant occurs with a vaginal delivery during a primary genital herpes simplex virus (HSV) infection. Infection most commonly occurs by direct transmission, rather than across the placenta. The risk of transmission during vaginal delivery with an active primary infection is approximately 50%. Neonates with symptomatic HSV infection are often critically ill and may suffer chronic complications as a result of the neonatal infection. Risk of transmission to the infant with vaginal delivery during an active secondary HSV infection drops significantly to less than 5%. Cesarean section is recommended for women with signs of an active primary or secondary genital HSV outbreak around the time of delivery. Transmission is low in patients with a history of genital HSV infection who have no signs or symptoms of an active outbreak around the time of delivery

102. B: Fetal heart rate variability reflects the interplay between cardiac responsiveness and the sympathetic and parasympathetic nervous systems. Baseline fetal heart variability refers to the degree of fluctuation in the fetal heart rate around the baseline. An amplitude of 6–25 beats/min in fetal heart rate variability (moderate variability) is considered normal. Decreased fetal heart rate variability is the best predictor of fetal compromise. Causes of decreased fetal heart rate variability include hypoxia, acidosis, gestational age under 32 weeks, fetal anomalies, central nervous system depressant medications, fetal tachycardia, and preexisting fetal neurologic abnormalities. Marked fetal heart rate variability of more than 25 beats/min amplitude (saltatory variability) is usually caused by early hypoxia, as occurs with umbilical cord compression, and is considered a nonreassuring pattern.

103. A: Precipitous labor is defined as labor that leads to delivery of the infant in less than 3 hours. A major predictive factor for precipitous labor is a history of previous precipitous labor. Precipitous labor may be anticipated if there is rapid cervical dilation, rapid fetal descent, or intense, frequent

uterine contractions. Maternal risks with precipitous labor include cervical, vaginal, and perineal injury; postpartum hemorrhage as a result of both lacerations and uterine atony; and unaccompanied precipitous delivery. Fetal risks include hypoxia secondary to uterine hypertonicity and brachial plexus injury as a result of rapid descent and delivery. Precipitous labor in the group B *Streptococcus*–positive patient may not allow adequate time for administration of prophylactic antibiotics.

104. C: When an Rh-negative patient is pregnant with an Rh-positive fetus, any maternal exposure to fetal Rh-positive blood (e.g., spontaneous or therapeutic abortion, antepartum hemorrhage, delivery) can lead to sensitization or production of Rh antibodies in the maternal circulation. When maternal exposure (and sensitization) to fetal blood occurs at the time of delivery, the first Rh-positive infant is not affected. Subsequent Rh-positive fetuses in the sensitized Rh-negative mother are affected (often severely) by the hemolysis that occurs when maternal Rh antibodies cross the placenta and destroy fetal red blood cells. Rh-negative fetuses are not affected as their blood cells do not have Rh antigen. Rh-negative pregnant patients (who have not been sensitized) are given RhoGAM (Rh immune globulin) to prevent sensitization when there is a reasonable likelihood of maternal exposure to Rh-positive fetal blood.

105. B: Decreased fetal movement has been associated with fetal distress and death. There is no established standard for a normal number of fetal movements in a given time period. As a general rule, four fetal movements in 1 hour or ten fetal movements in 2 hours is considered reassuring. If a patient reports decreased fetal movement over the preceding hour she should be instructed to have something to eat or drink, lie on her left side, and count fetal movements over the next 1-2 hours. Patterns of fetal movement are dependent on multiple factors, including time of day, location of the placenta, maternal medications, and the fetal sleep cycle. Low-risk patients reporting decreased fetal movement of less than 2–3 hours duration can be instructed to count fetal movements and inform the health care provider if there are less than ten movements in 2 hours (after 32–34 weeks' gestation). It has not been definitively demonstrated that prompt evaluation of decreased fetal movement results in improved fetal outcomes.

106. B: Neonatal anemia may result from blood loss (placental abruption, placenta previa, internal hemorrhage, blood draws), increased destruction of red blood cells (hereditary blood disorders, immune hemolysis [Rh/ABO incompatibility]), or decreased production of red blood cells (anemia of prematurity, bone marrow suppression, iron deficiency anemia). Mild anemia may be asymptomatic. Symptoms with severe anemia include pallor, tachypnea, hypotension, tachycardia, apnea, metabolic acidosis, jaundice, and poor feeding. Treatment includes limiting blood draws, treating underlying cause, and partial exchange transfusions with PRBCs (for severe cases). Hematocrit below 45% at term indicates anemia.

Weeks gestation	Hemoglobin	Hematocrit	Reticulocyte count
37 to term	16.8 g/dL	53%	3-7%
32	15 g/dL	47%	3-10%
28 weeks	14.5	45%	5-10%

107. A: Although each patient's labor and delivery are unique, there are features that are common to the different stages of labor and delivery in many patients. The first stage of labor (from onset of active labor to complete cervical dilation) is divided into latent, active, and transition phases. The latent phase starts with the beginning of regular contractions and ends when the cervix is 3 cm dilated. Patients are often talkative and coping well in this stage. The active phase occurs as the cervix dilates to 7 cm and as patients become more uncomfortable, focused, and potentially more anxious. The transition phase encompasses the final several centimeters of cervical dilation (8–10

cm). Contractions during transition are more frequent and intense; patients are often restless, irritable, and nauseated and feel growing rectal pressure as the fetus descends.

108. B: The nurse must always treat the patient, not the monitor. Before intervention, put eyes on the mother and assess both mother and fetus to rule out artifact. Artifacts and signal ambiguity should be suspected when the fetal heart rates continue at a low normal rate, at least 50% of contractions result in accelerations of FHR, and the FHR appears to decelerate to the maternal heart rate and does not return to baseline. If signal ambiguity is expected, the maternal pulse rate should be counted and traced and fetal and maternal tracings compared.

109. A: The definitive indication of true labor is progressive cervical change. It can be difficult to distinguish between true and false labor in the absence of a cervical exam. In general, the uterine contractions of false labor occur at irregular intervals and do not progressively increase in duration or intensity. By definition, the contractions of false labor are not associated with progressive cervical change. The pain associated with false labor is usually concentrated in the groin and anterior abdomen, while true labor pain often begins in the back and radiates to the abdominal region. Rest or a warm bath often decrease the contractions of false labor but do not relieve the contractions associated with true labor.

110. C: Face presentation results in the fetal head being hyperextended, rather than flexed, as the infant is delivered. Face presentation results in a significantly larger presenting part during vaginal delivery, which increases the likelihood of cephalopelvic disproportion and prolonged or stalled labor. Trauma to the face as the fetus passes through the pelvis leads to an increased risk of neonatal facial edema. Newborns delivered in face presentation are also more likely to have respiratory distress (as a result of laryngeal edema), nonreassuring fetal status, and intrapartum death. If the chin is posterior and remains in that position, cesarean delivery is necessary. Attempts to rotate the fetus in face presentation are associated with higher rates of both maternal and fetal complications (including death) and are, therefore, contraindicated

111. B: Nurses are not immune to drug and alcohol dependence. The easy access to controlled substances in combination with the nurse's responsibility for the health and safety of patients makes prompt intervention for the impaired nurse absolutely critical. The impaired nurse may be diverting drugs that should either be "wasted" or administered to the patient. Staff members should be educated about the signs of substance abuse and counseled to report any concern about nurse impairment immediately to the appropriate supervisor. Most institutions offer substance abuse counseling and resources to the impaired nurse with established policies for returning to patient care when appropriate.

112. B: Mongolian spots (congenital dermal melanocytosis) are blue-gray, nontender, irregular discolorations typically present at birth. They are due to entrapment of melanocytes in the dermis and are most often seen in the lumbosacral region. Mongolian spots are most commonly seen in newborns of African-American, Asian, Hispanic, and Native American descent. Mongolian spots appear similar to bruises and may be mistaken for signs of birth trauma. Bruises from birth trauma are unusual in the region of the flank and buttocks. Erythema toxicum is a benign newborn rash that typically appears 1–2 days after birth and consists of small, yellow papules on a flat red base.

113. A: At least 20% of pregnant patients are estimated to be affected by domestic violence during pregnancy. Unfortunately, incidents of domestic violence often increase in frequency during pregnancy, particularly in cases involving pregnant adolescents or unwanted pregnancies. Physical assaults during pregnancy more commonly involve the genital, abdominal, and breast regions than abuse that occurs in the nonpregnant patient. Complications resulting from abuse of the pregnant

patient include bleeding, insufficient weight gain, preterm labor, placental abruption, fetal death, visceral injury in intra-abdominal organs (e.g., spleen, liver, uterus), fetal injury, and infection. The emotional toll of partner abuse is an additional complication for both the pregnant woman and her fetus or infant.

114. B: Psychosocial and cultural assessment of the obstetrical patient in active labor is a critical evaluation tool that is included in the initial patient assessment and continues as labor and delivery progress. Key components of the psychosocial and cultural assessment of the obstetrical patient include evaluation of the patient's beliefs and preferences about the childbirth process; knowledge, fears, and expectations; plans for pain relief; and preexisting psychosocial challenges that may affect the patient's labor experience. Ongoing assessment of the patient's pain management strategies, anxiety, and coping skills is important as frequently patients require variable levels of psychosocial support as labor progresses or unexpected complications develop.

115. B: Labor is described as occurring in four stages. The first stage of labor starts with the onset of true labor (uterine contractions resulting in progressive cervical change) and ends with complete cervical dilation to 10 cm. The first stage of labor can be divided into latent, active, and transition phases. The second stage of labor starts with compete cervical dilation and ends when the newborn is delivered. The third stage of labor begins after delivery of the infant and ends with delivery of the placenta. The fourth stage of labor occurs in the several hours after delivery of the placenta when post-delivery physiologic adjustments occur in the postpartum patient.

116. A: Intrauterine resuscitation refers to clinical interventions aimed at improving fetal well-being and are often undertaken in response to nonreassuring fetal heart rate patterns. Diagnostic maneuvers in response to nonreassuring fetal heart rate tracings should include assessment for cord prolapse, rapid fetal descent, rapid cervical dilation, uterine hyperstimulation, maternal infection, and maternal hypotension. Therapeutic maneuvers aimed at improving fetal well-being can then be tailored to the specific clinical situation. Common interventions in response to nonreassuring fetal heart rate patterns include changes in maternal position (usually to left lateral or right lateral position to improve uterine blood flow), intravenous fluid administration to optimize uteroplacental perfusion or to correct maternal hypotension, and high-flow oxygen administration to improve fetal oxygen delivery. Other interventions may include amnioinfusion to decrease umbilical cord compression, reduction of uterine activity (e.g., tocolytic administration or reduction in oxytocin administration), and an alteration or reduction in pushing efforts. In all cases of nonreassuring fetal status, staff must be prepared for emergent operative delivery.

117. B: Amniotic fluid embolism (AFE) is fortunately a rare complication of pregnancy, but it carries a significant risk of chronic neurologic disability and death in the mother. Possible risk factors for AFE include male fetus, advanced maternal age, and multiparity, although AFE is essentially an unpredictable complication. Most commonly AFE occurs during labor or in the immediate postpartum period but may also occur with cesarean delivery, abdominal trauma, or abortion; it can present in dramatic fashion with respiratory distress or arrest, cardiovascular collapse, mental status changes, seizures, and massive coagulopathy with hemorrhage (disseminated intravascular coagulation). Treatment is supportive, including respiratory and hemodynamic support and treatment of coagulopathy. Many patients die within 1 hour of onset, and prompt cesarean delivery of the fetus is indicated in cases where the mother cannot be resuscitated.

118. C: One of the important ongoing assessments during labor is evaluation of the frequency, duration, and intensity of uterine contractions. The nurse can place one hand on the uterine fundus and assess all three factors. The frequency of contractions is evaluated by noting the time from the start of one contraction until the start of the next contraction. The duration of contractions is

- 138 -

evaluated by noting the start and end time of a single contraction. As the first stage of labor progresses, contractions become more frequent and last longer. The intensity of contractions can also be assessed with fundal palpation. During the peak of a contraction, fundal indentability is assessed. The stronger the contraction, the less indentable the uterine fundus is.

119. C: External cephalic version (ECV) of the fetus in breech presentation consists of external manipulation of the fetus into a cephalic position. Candidates for ECV attempts should have an ultrasound-confirmed breech or transverse presentation, reassuring fetal status (reactive nonstress test) before the procedure, and a gestational age of at least 36 weeks. Contraindications to attempted external version include any condition that precludes a vaginal delivery (e.g., placenta previa, active genital herpes infection); nonreassuring fetal status; multiple gestation; uterine, fetal, or amniotic fluid abnormality; or previous significant uterine surgery, including cesarean section. Rh-negative status is not a contraindication to ECV, but RhoGAM should be administered after the procedure. Complications include fetal compromise or injury, placental abruption, and premature rupture of membranes. Fetal heart rate should be monitored before, during, and after attempted version.

120. C: Maternal hypotension is the most common side effect of epidural anesthesia, occurring in up to one-third of patients. Hypotension occurs because the nerve fibers that regulate vasodilation are anesthetized. Maternal hypotension can lead to impaired uterine blood flow and fetal hypoxia. Maternal and fetal status in the patient receiving epidural anesthesia must be monitored closely, and the nurse should be ready to intervene if the patient becomes hypotensive. Immediate management includes administration of an intravenous fluid bolus and oxygen and left lateral positioning. Vasopressors (e.g., ephedrine) may be required if hypotension is not responsive to those measures. Other common complications of epidural anesthesia include urinary retention, back pain, and headache in the case of accidental dural puncture.

121. C: Induction of labor is defined as stimulation of uterine contractions before the onset of spontaneous labor. Cervical readiness is the most important factor in the prediction of successful labor induction and is most commonly assessed, using the Bishop scoring system. The higher the overall score (corresponding to a more favorable cervix), the more likely labor induction will be successful. Factors assessed and scored are the degree of cervical dilation, effacement, consistency, and position in addition to fetal station. Methods used for induction of labor include oxytocin administration, amniotomy (artificial rupture of membranes), and manually stripping the amniotic membranes. Many patients use alternative methods of labor induction, such as nipple stimulation, sexual intercourse, and acupuncture.

122. A: A patient presenting late in pregnancy with painless, bright red vaginal bleeding needs to be evaluated for placenta previa, where the placenta is implanted in the lower uterine segment and either partially or completely covering the cervical os. A digital vaginal exam is absolutely contraindicated in this clinical setting until placenta previa has been ruled out because it can cause life-threatening hemorrhage in these patients. Sterile speculum exam is not contraindicated and may be part of the initial evaluation. Transvaginal or transabdominal ultrasonographic evaluation is the initial study of choice for the evaluation of late-pregnancy vaginal bleeding. Risk factors for placenta previa include prior cesarean delivery, advanced maternal age, and maternal cigarette smoking. Complete placenta previa is an absolute contraindication to vaginal delivery

123. A: Newborn infants have several characteristics that impair their ability to avoid heat loss: a limited shivering capacity, a large body surface area relative to body mass, and a limited amount of subcutaneous fat. Newborns lose heat to their environment by four mechanisms. (1) Evaporative heat loss occurs when the fluid on the newborn's skin (e.g., amniotic fluid) is converted to vapor;

Copyright © Mometrix Media. You have been licensed one copy of this document for personal use only. Any other reproduction or redistribution is strictly prohibited. All rights reserved.

drying the infant after delivery minimizes heat lost through evaporation. (2) Convective heat loss occurs when heat is lost to cool air passing over the infant's skin; clothing the infant, maintaining warm room temperature, and eliminating drafts minimize heat lost through convection. (3) Heat loss via radiation occurs when heat is transferred from the warm infant to a nearby cool surface (not in direct contact with the infant), such as windows or isolette walls. (4) Finally, heat loss through conduction occurs when heat is lost from the warm infant directly to a cool surface (in direct contact with the infant), such as cold hands, stethoscope, or blankets; skin-to-skin contact between the mother and infant helps to prevent conductive heat loss, as well as enhance the mother–infant attachment.

124. B: Determination of fetal lung maturity is important in decisions involving elective near-term delivery or timing of planned delivery for patients with pregnancy complications (e.g., hypertension, preeclampsia) so that iatrogenic complications of prematurity can be avoided. Determination of fetal lung maturity is essentially an assessment of whether there is adequate surfactant being produced by the fetal lungs to stabilize and maintain open pulmonary alveoli during spontaneous breathing in the neonate. Lecithin and sphingomyelin are components of surfactant, which can be measured in amniotic fluid. A lecithin/sphingomyelin (L/S) ratio of at least 2:1 indicates fetal lung maturity. Phosphatidylglycerol is another component of surfactant; its presence indicates fetal lung maturity, and its detection is unaffected by amniotic fluid contaminated with blood or meconium.

125. B: Forceps are used during vaginal delivery to assist with rotation of the malpositioned fetus into an occiput-anterior position or to expedite the second stage of delivery if there are maternal or fetal complications requiring urgent delivery. Forceps should only be used if the membranes are ruptured, cervical dilation is complete, the fetal head is engaged, and adequate anesthesia is provided. Forceps are placed by an experienced medical provider, and traction is applied during contractions as the patient pushes. Traction is not generally applied between contractions. Complications of forceps-assisted delivery include perineal lacerations in the mother and facial lacerations, bruising, and brachial plexus injuries in the infant.

126. A: The most common type of uterine incision with cesarean section is the low transverse uterine incision. This type of incision involves less blood loss than vertical uterine incisions, is easier to repair, and is less likely to rupture during subsequent pregnancies. Disadvantages of the low transverse uterine incision include longer time to delivery of the infant and limited incision size due to proximity of major uterine vessels. The most common alternative to the low transverse uterine incision is the low uterine segment vertical incision. This type of incision is preferred for multiple gestations, anterior placental previa, fetal distress, preterm delivery (as a result of a poorly formed lower uterine segment), and macrosomic fetuses. Blood loss is greater, and repair is more difficult with the vertical incision. Extension of the incision into the more contractile, upper portion of the uterus is associated with a marked increase in the risk of uterine rupture with subsequent pregnancies (even without labor).

127. B: Intrapartum fetal heart rate monitoring requires documentation and interpretation of five variables: baseline fetal heart rate, heart rate variability, presence or absence of fetal heart rate accelerations, fetal heart rate decelerations and their relation to uterine contractions, and changes in the fetal heart rate pattern as labor progresses. A reassuring fetal heart tracing should demonstrate a baseline heart rate between 110–160 beats/min with accelerations, moderate variability, and the absence of late or variable decelerations (early decelerations may be observed). Any deviation from these variables constitutes an indeterminate or nonreassuring pattern that requires further evaluation and management as indicated. Ominous fetal heart rate patterns

requiring immediate intervention or delivery include sinusoidal patterns, prolonged severe bradycardia, and persistent variable or late decelerations with loss of variability.

128. A: Engorgement is characterized by bilateral breast pain, warmth, and firm texture; it is often difficult for the breastfeeding infant to latch onto engorged breasts. Patients with a plugged milk duct have unilateral, localized pain in the region of the plugged duct, often with a palpable firm lump in the affected area. Neither engorgement nor plugged milk ducts are usually associated with systemic signs of illness, such as fever or flu-like symptoms. In contrast, mastitis presents with focal, unilateral breast pain with a warm, red, and tender region of the affected breast and accompanying signs of systemic illness. Mastitis typically occurs when bacteria from the infant's mouth or mother's skin ascends through a traumatized nipple. Treatment includes frequent breastfeeding, pain relievers, and systemic antibiotics.

129. B: Shoulder dystocia during a vaginal delivery is recognized when the usual technique for delivering the fetal shoulders is unsuccessful (prolonged head-to-body birth interval). The "turtle sign" may occur, when the fetal head retracts against the perineum after emerging. A common mnemonic for maneuvers that are used to relieve shoulder dystocia is HELPERR: H (call for **h**elp), E (consider **e**pisiotomy), L (**l**egs into the knee–chest position or the McRoberts maneuver, P (suprapubic **p**ressure), E (**e**nter maneuvers where the medical provider inserts his or her hand into the vagina to rotate the fetal shoulders into a deliverable position), R (**r**emove posterior arm = delivery of posterior arm), and R (**r**oll patient onto hands and knees). Application of fundal pressure will likely worsen impaction of the fetal shoulder. If these maneuvers are unsuccessful, providers may push the fetal head back into the vagina and proceed to emergent cesarean delivery.

130. C: Preterm labor is defined as uterine contractions that lead to cervical change between 20 and 36 weeks of pregnancy. Preterm labor and preterm birth rates have increased over the last several decades. Neonatal rates of respiratory distress syndrome, intraventricular hemorrhage, necrotizing enterocolitis, and death progressively increase with lower gestational age. In the absence of chorioamnionitis, patients in preterm labor should receive corticosteroids. Steroid administration in patients with preterm labor is associated with a decreased risk for neonatal respiratory distress syndrome and mortality. Typically, two doses of either betamethasone or dexamethasone are administered intramuscularly in the patient with preterm labor and no signs of chorioamnionitis.

131. C: Changes during pregnancy increase the risk of thromboembolic disease in all pregnant patients as a result of a variety of physiologic factors (e.g., relative increase in pro-coagulation and increased venous stasis). Multiple factors increase the pregnant patient's risk for thromboembolic disease, including advanced maternal age, obesity, immobility, operative delivery, dehydration, and extremity trauma, including injury from inadequate padding of pressure points or a prolonged period in stirrups during labor. Early ambulation after delivery and adequate fluid intake can reduce the risk of postpartum thromboembolic complications.

132. A: Patients receiving oxytocin for labor induction or augmentation need to be closely monitored for signs of uterine hyperstimulation, which may be accompanied by signs of fetal compromise. A productive contraction frequency and intensity will lead to 1 cm/hr of cervical change during active labor. Contractions that occur every 2–3 minutes, last 40–60 seconds, and are of moderate intensity are generally considered "adequate" during labor augmentation, although cervical change remains the ultimate determinant of productive contractions. Oxytocin administration can lead to hypercontractility of the uterus, which can lead to placental abruption; fetal hypoxia as a result of impaired uterine blood flow; uterine rupture; and precipitous delivery. Signs of a hyperstimulated uterus include contractions occurring more frequently than every 2 minutes and lasting longer than 60 seconds and increased uterine tone between contractions.

Management of uterine hyperstimulation with signs of fetal compromise includes immediate discontinuation of oxytocin, intravenous fluid administration, maternal repositioning onto the left side, and oxygen administration.

133. C: Fetal scalp stimulation is a relatively noninvasive, quick way to assess fetal well-being in the presence of nonreassuring fetal heart rate monitoring patterns and may reduce the need for more invasive evaluations like fetal scalp blood sampling. A medical provider applies pressure to the fetal scalp or massages the fetal scalp for 15 seconds during a digital vaginal exam. Fetal heart rate accelerations of 15 beats/min or more above baseline and lasting for 15 seconds or more in response to fetal scalp stimulation have been shown to correlate well with a nonacidotic fetus.

134. B: Poorly controlled diabetes mellitus during pregnancy leads to a number of complications for the fetus and newborn infant. Maternal hyperglycemia leads to fetal hyperglycemia as glucose freely crosses the placenta into the fetal circulation. Fetal insulin production increases in response to the hyperglycemia, leading to excessive fetal growth (in most cases). Infants of diabetic mothers are often hypoglycemic soon after birth as a result of the presence of elevated insulin levels (despite no further exposure to the hyperglycemia of the maternal circulation). Other common complications in the infant of a diabetic mother include birth trauma (due to macrosomia), polycythemia, hypocalcemia, congenital anomalies, and respiratory distress syndrome. Maternal diabetes that is associated with chronic vascular complications may lead to intrauterine growth restriction as a result of placental insufficiency.

135. C: Almost one-third of deliveries in the United States are by cesarean birth. Common indications for cesarean delivery include placenta previa/abruption, active genital herpes infection, nonreassuring fetal status, fetal malposition, prior cesarean delivery, and labor dystocia (e.g., failure to progress). Cesarean delivery is associated with an increased risk of multiple maternal and fetal complications, including increased maternal mortality, surgical wound infections, fetal respiratory distress, and admissions to the neonatal intensive care unit. Women who have undergone cesarean delivery have an increased risk of placental complications in subsequent pregnancies, including abruption and previa. Women in the postpartum period who have undergone cesarean delivery usually require a higher level of support and assistance with newborn care as a result of postoperative pain, limited mobility, and side effects from pain medications. Women who have cesarean delivery often do not experience damage to the pelvic floor associated with vaginal delivery that can lead to future incontinence.

136. A: Umbilical cord prolapse is a true obstetrical emergency and poses a significant risk to the fetus. Umbilical cord prolapse may be overt (palpable or visibly prolapsed through the cervix ahead of the presenting fetal part) or occult (alongside the presenting fetal part). Nonreassuring fetal status in the patient with ruptured membranes should prompt a vaginal exam to evaluate for umbilical cord prolapse. This includes a deterioration in fetal status after artificial rupture of membranes. Cord prolapse results in fetal compromise because of an impaired umbilical blood flow as a result of mechanical compression or vasospasm. Management includes minimal handling of the umbilical cord, maternal Trendelenburg or deep knee–chest position to reduce cord compression, intravaginal elevation of the presenting fetal part, and imminent delivery. Vaginal birth may be indicated if the cervix is completely dilated and delivery is imminent.

137. C: Polycythemia (venous hematocrit over 65%) of the newborn usually occurs in response to either fetal hypoxia or intrauterine transfusion. Risk factors for polycythemia include placental insufficiency (e.g., preeclampsia, maternal hypertension, post-term), poorly controlled gestational diabetes, delayed umbilical cord clamping, twin–twin transfusion, maternal cigarette smoking, and certain chromosomal disorders (e.g., trisomy 21, 13, and 18). Polycythemia rarely occurs in infants

- 142 -

born before 34 weeks' gestation. Polycythemia may lead to hyperviscosity, which leads to impaired tissue perfusion. Signs of symptomatic polycythemia in the newborn include lethargy, irritability, poor feeding, respiratory distress, apnea, ruddy skin tone, oliguria, hypoglycemia, and hypocalcemia. Treatment of symptomatic infants is with partial exchange transfusion.

138. A: Tocolytics are medications used for the purpose of arresting preterm labor, although they appear to be most useful for delaying preterm birth by 1–2 days rather than arresting preterm labor until term. Common tocolytic medications include beta-agonists (e.g., terbutaline), magnesium sulfate, calcium channel blockers (e.g., nifedipine), and prostaglandin inhibitors (e.g., indomethacin). Tocolysis of preterm labor is contraindicated in the presence of fetal distress, severe preeclampsia or eclampsia, uncontrolled gestational diabetes, intra-amniotic infection, significant maternal cardiac or pulmonary disease, maternal hemodynamic instability, and fetal demise. Specific tocolytic agents are contraindicated in other clinical situations as well. Other contraindications include the fetus weight being less than 2500 grams or cervix dilation being more than 4 cm.

139. B: One of the most effective nonpharmacologic pain management techniques during labor and delivery is maternal repositioning to the position of maximum comfort. One of the disadvantages of the modern labor and delivery experience is the limitation in maternal position or movement to the recumbent lithotomy position. Although this position allows for easier maternal and fetal monitoring and perineal access, it has a number of disadvantages, including a higher rate of labor dystocia, maternal discomfort, and perineal trauma during delivery. When possible, patients in labor should be encouraged to try out a number of different positions to find the one most comfortable for them as labor progresses.

140. B: Proper and thorough education regarding common symptoms and warning signs for both the postpartum patient and her newborn infant is important before hospital discharge. This should include breast-feeding techniques and complications, perineal care, signs of infection or hemorrhage, expected emotional changes, dietary needs, basic infant care, and signs of illness in the infant. Signs and symptoms that should be reported promptly to a health care provider include fever; foul-smelling lochia; increasing wound, perineal, abdominal, or breast pain; signs of thromboembolic disease; excessive bleeding; and severe postpartum depression or psychosis. Foul-smelling lochia may indicate endometritis. Hemorrhoids are a common postpartum complication, which often resolve within weeks of delivery. Uterine cramps with breast-feeding are common as a result of the release of oxytocin at the initiation of a breast-feeding session.

141. B: Factors associated with higher success rates of vaginal birth after prior cesarean (VBAC) include spontaneous labor, prior vaginal delivery, favorable cervix, and no use of cervical ripening (prostaglandin) or labor induction agents (oxytocin). Factors associated with lower success rates include fetal macrosomia, maternal obesity, history of labor dystocia, and gestational age over 41 weeks. The risk for uterine rupture is elevated in patients attempting VBAC, and the risk increases with the use of labor induction or cervical ripening agents, a history of vertical uterine incision, a short interval since the last pregnancy, a history of single-layer uterine closure, or a history of infection with prior cesarean. A VBAC should only be attempted in a facility where there is immediate availability of full surgical and neonatal teams in the event of uterine rupture or other life-threatening complication.

142. B: Hypothyroidism (particularly severe, untreated hypothyroidism) in the pregnant patient is associated with an increased risk of fetal loss and abnormalities in fetal brain development. In the first trimester of pregnancy, maternal thyroid hormone crosses the placenta in significant amounts and is critical for normal fetal brain development. Maternal hypothyroidism is also associated with

an increased risk of neonatal hypothyroidism, although most cases of congenital hypothyroidism are secondary to factors independent of maternal thyroid status during pregnancy.

143. A: Systemic lupus erythematosus in the pregnant patient poses a risk for both the mother and fetus, particularly in the patient who has active, symptomatic lupus. Pregnant women with lupus have an increased incidence of renal disease, preeclampsia, urinary tract infection, gestational diabetes, thrombosis, and premature rupture of membranes. Risk of intrauterine fetal demise is markedly increased in pregnancies complicated by maternal lupus. Although neonatal lupus is uncommon, it typically presents with either a characteristic lupus rash or congenital heart block. Specific lupus-associated antibodies are linked with specific fetal and neonatal complications.

144. C: Premature rupture of membranes (PROM) is defined as rupture of membranes before labor begins, while rupture of membranes without labor before 37 weeks is referred to as preterm premature rupture of membranes (PPROM). Pregnant patients with PROM may present with leaking fluid, vaginal discharge, pelvic pressure, or vaginal bleeding. Confirmation of membrane rupture may be performed by visualizing pooled fluid in the vagina on sterile speculum exam, nitrazine paper testing, examination for "ferning" of fluid, or ultrasound. Complications of PROM include chorioamnionitis, placental abruption, fetal/neonatal sepsis, malpresentation, umbilical cord prolapse, and complications related to prematurity if membrane rupture occurs before 37 weeks' gestation. Digital vaginal exams should be minimized because of an increased infection risk. Providers and patients may opt for expectant management of PROM at term as most patients will have spontaneous labor within 24 hours of membrane rupture. Rupture of membranes longer than 24 hours before delivery markedly increases the risk of infection.

145. B: Multiple gestation pregnancies are considered high-risk in all cases as a result of the increase in maternal and fetal complications. Maternal complications include an elevated risk of anemia, preeclampsia, gestational diabetes, hyperemesis gravidarum, hypertension, preterm labor, amniotic fluid embolism, cesarean delivery, antepartum and postpartum hemorrhage, endometritis, cholestasis, peripartum cardiomyopathy, and maternal death. Fetal and neonatal complications include increased risk for intrauterine growth restriction, discordant growth, twin–twin transfusion syndrome, congenital anomalies, malpresentation, cord prolapse, preterm delivery, and fetal death. Both maternal polycythemia and post-term delivery are less common in multiple gestation pregnancies.

146. A: Risks to the hypertensive pregnant patient include abruption, seizures, renal failure, cardiac failure, pulmonary edema, and intracerebral hemorrhage. Hypertension is associated with placental insufficiency, leading to intrauterine growth restriction, oligohydramnios, and increased risk of fetal death. In general, hypertension associated with preeclampsia (with or without concurrent chronic, preexisting hypertension) is associated with greater risk to both the fetus and mother. Pregnancy-induced hypertension (PIH) is defined as hypertension that develops after 20 weeks' gestation, is not associated with signs of preeclampsia, and resolves in the postpartum period. Outcomes are generally good for both mother and fetus as long as the PIH does not progress to preeclampsia.

147. A: Although use of continuous fetal heart rate (FHR) monitoring is extremely common in the hospital setting, there is no definitive evidence of its benefit in low-risk patients; its use is associated with an increased likelihood of cesarean and instrumented delivery. Continuous FHR monitoring is indicated, however, when the risk of fetal hypoxia is increased due to maternal or fetal complications or medical interventions during labor. Clinical situations where continuous external FHR monitoring is indicated include preeclampsia, placenta previa or abruption, multiple gestation, preterm labor, induction of labor, nonreassuring fetal status, maternal fever, and

congenital malformations. If assessing FHR intermittently, low-risk patients should have FHR auscultated every 30 minutes during the first stage of labor and every 15 minutes during the second stage of labor. High-risk patients should have FHR auscultated every 15 minutes during the first stage of labor and every 5 minutes during the second stage.

148. C: Early fetal heart rate decelerations are caused by a vagal response to compression of the fetal head with uterine contractions. Early decelerations have a gradual onset coinciding with the onset of a contraction and gradual resolution coinciding with the end of the contraction. The waveform of early decelerations often looks like a mirror image of the contraction waveform. Early fetal heart rate decelerations are not associated with fetal compromise and do not require intervention. This is in contrast to late decelerations, which are usually caused by uteroplacental insufficiency, and variable decelerations, which are caused by umbilical cord compression.

149. B: Abruptio placentae (placental abruption) is characterized by premature separation of the placenta from its site of implantation, usually in the latter half of pregnancy. Placental abruption accounts for about 15% of fetal and neonatal deaths. Risk factors for placental abruption include maternal hypertension (the most common associated factor), trauma, preterm premature rupture of membranes, and maternal cocaine abuse. Depending on the location and degree of placental abruption, vaginal bleeding may be absent or deceptively minimal relative to the extent of bleeding. Unlike placenta previa, placental abruption is usually accompanied by uterine pain and tenderness. Other clinical features of placental abruption include abnormal uterine tone/contractions, fetal distress, and maternal signs of hemorrhagic shock. Placenta accreta (abnormal implantation of the placenta directly into the myometrium) presents during the third stage of labor with abnormal or incomplete placental separation and may be accompanied by significant postpartum hemorrhage and uterine atony.

150. C: Amniocentesis is performed by inserting a needle through the pregnant patient's abdomen to obtain a sample of amniotic fluid, using ultrasound guidance to minimize the risk of puncturing the placenta, umbilical cord, or fetus. Amniocentesis is generally performed either to screen for genetic abnormalities in the fetus (e.g., spina bifida, trisomy 21) or evaluate fetal lung maturity. Patients undergoing amniocentesis have an increased risk of miscarriage, infection, premature rupture of membranes, and accidental puncture of the placenta, cord, or fetus. Patients are instructed to avoid strenuous activity or sexual intercourse for 1–2 days after the procedure. The medical provider should be notified about signs of infection at the puncture site, fever, abnormal fetal movement, significant cramping, and persistent or heavy vaginal bleeding or discharge

How to Overcome Test Anxiety

Just the thought of taking a test is enough to make most people a little nervous. A test is an important event that can have a long-term impact on your future, so it's important to take it seriously and it's natural to feel anxious about performing well. But just because anxiety is normal, that doesn't mean that it's helpful in test taking, or that you should simply accept it as part of your life. Anxiety can have a variety of effects. These effects can be mild, like making you feel slightly nervous, or severe, like blocking your ability to focus or remember even a simple detail.

If you experience test anxiety—whether severe or mild—it's important to know how to beat it. To discover this, first you need to understand what causes test anxiety.

Causes of Test Anxiety

While we often think of anxiety as an uncontrollable emotional state, it can actually be caused by simple, practical things. One of the most common causes of test anxiety is that a person does not feel adequately prepared for their test. This feeling can be the result of many different issues such as poor study habits or lack of organization, but the most common culprit is time management. Starting to study too late, failing to organize your study time to cover all of the material, or being distracted while you study will mean that you're not well prepared for the test. This may lead to cramming the night before, which will cause you to be physically and mentally exhausted for the test. Poor time management also contributes to feelings of stress, fear, and hopelessness as you realize you are not well prepared but don't know what to do about it.

Other times, test anxiety is not related to your preparation for the test but comes from unresolved fear. This may be a past failure on a test, or poor performance on tests in general. It may come from comparing yourself to others who seem to be performing better or from the stress of living up to expectations. Anxiety may be driven by fears of the future—how failure on this test would affect your educational and career goals. These fears are often completely irrational, but they can still negatively impact your test performance.

> **Review Video:** <u>3 Reasons You Have Test Anxiety</u>
> Visit mometrix.com/academy and enter code: 428468

Elements of Test Anxiety

As mentioned earlier, test anxiety is considered to be an emotional state, but it has physical and mental components as well. Sometimes you may not even realize that you are suffering from test anxiety until you notice the physical symptoms. These can include trembling hands, rapid heartbeat, sweating, nausea, and tense muscles. Extreme anxiety may lead to fainting or vomiting. Obviously, any of these symptoms can have a negative impact on testing. It is important to recognize them as soon as they begin to occur so that you can address the problem before it damages your performance.

> **Review Video:** 3 Ways to Tell You Have Test Anxiety
> Visit mometrix.com/academy and enter code: 927847

The mental components of test anxiety include trouble focusing and inability to remember learned information. During a test, your mind is on high alert, which can help you recall information and stay focused for an extended period of time. However, anxiety interferes with your mind's natural processes, causing you to blank out, even on the questions you know well. The strain of testing during anxiety makes it difficult to stay focused, especially on a test that may take several hours. Extreme anxiety can take a huge mental toll, making it difficult not only to recall test information but even to understand the test questions or pull your thoughts together.

> **Review Video:** How Test Anxiety Affects Memory
> Visit mometrix.com/academy and enter code: 609003

Effects of Test Anxiety

Test anxiety is like a disease—if left untreated, it will get progressively worse. Anxiety leads to poor performance, and this reinforces the feelings of fear and failure, which in turn lead to poor performances on subsequent tests. It can grow from a mild nervousness to a crippling condition. If allowed to progress, test anxiety can have a big impact on your schooling, and consequently on your future.

Test anxiety can spread to other parts of your life. Anxiety on tests can become anxiety in any stressful situation, and blanking on a test can turn into panicking in a job situation. But fortunately, you don't have to let anxiety rule your testing and determine your grades. There are a number of relatively simple steps you can take to move past anxiety and function normally on a test and in the rest of life.

> **Review Video:** How Test Anxiety Impacts Your Grades
> Visit mometrix.com/academy and enter code: 939819

Physical Steps for Beating Test Anxiety

While test anxiety is a serious problem, the good news is that it can be overcome. It doesn't have to control your ability to think and remember information. While it may take time, you can begin taking steps today to beat anxiety.

Just as your first hint that you may be struggling with anxiety comes from the physical symptoms, the first step to treating it is also physical. Rest is crucial for having a clear, strong mind. If you are tired, it is much easier to give in to anxiety. But if you establish good sleep habits, your body and mind will be ready to perform optimally, without the strain of exhaustion. Additionally, sleeping well helps you to retain information better, so you're more likely to recall the answers when you see the test questions.

Getting good sleep means more than going to bed on time. It's important to allow your brain time to relax. Take study breaks from time to time so it doesn't get overworked, and don't study right before bed. Take time to rest your mind before trying to rest your body, or you may find it difficult to fall asleep.

> **Review Video:** <u>The Importance of Sleep for Your Brain</u>
> Visit mometrix.com/academy and enter code: 319338

Along with sleep, other aspects of physical health are important in preparing for a test. Good nutrition is vital for good brain function. Sugary foods and drinks may give a burst of energy but this burst is followed by a crash, both physically and emotionally. Instead, fuel your body with protein and vitamin-rich foods.

Also, drink plenty of water. Dehydration can lead to headaches and exhaustion, especially if your brain is already under stress from the rigors of the test. Particularly if your test is a long one, drink water during the breaks. And if possible, take an energy-boosting snack to eat between sections.

> **Review Video:** <u>How Diet Can Affect your Mood</u>
> Visit mometrix.com/academy and enter code: 624317

Along with sleep and diet, a third important part of physical health is exercise. Maintaining a steady workout schedule is helpful, but even taking 5-minute study breaks to walk can help get your blood pumping faster and clear your head. Exercise also releases endorphins, which contribute to a positive feeling and can help combat test anxiety.

When you nurture your physical health, you are also contributing to your mental health. If your body is healthy, your mind is much more likely to be healthy as well. So take time to rest, nourish your body with healthy food and water, and get moving as much as possible. Taking these physical steps will make you stronger and more able to take the mental steps necessary to overcome test anxiety.

> **Review Video:** <u>How to Stay Healthy and Prevent Test Anxiety</u>
> Visit mometrix.com/academy and enter code: 877894

Mental Steps for Beating Test Anxiety

Working on the mental side of test anxiety can be more challenging, but as with the physical side, there are clear steps you can take to overcome it. As mentioned earlier, test anxiety often stems from lack of preparation, so the obvious solution is to prepare for the test. Effective studying may be the most important weapon you have for beating test anxiety, but you can and should employ several other mental tools to combat fear.

First, boost your confidence by reminding yourself of past success—tests or projects that you aced. If you're putting as much effort into preparing for this test as you did for those, there's no reason you should expect to fail here. Work hard to prepare; then trust your preparation.

Second, surround yourself with encouraging people. It can be helpful to find a study group, but be sure that the people you're around will encourage a positive attitude. If you spend time with others who are anxious or cynical, this will only contribute to your own anxiety. Look for others who are motivated to study hard from a desire to succeed, not from a fear of failure.

Third, reward yourself. A test is physically and mentally tiring, even without anxiety, and it can be helpful to have something to look forward to. Plan an activity following the test, regardless of the outcome, such as going to a movie or getting ice cream.

When you are taking the test, if you find yourself beginning to feel anxious, remind yourself that you know the material. Visualize successfully completing the test. Then take a few deep, relaxing breaths and return to it. Work through the questions carefully but with confidence, knowing that you are capable of succeeding.

Developing a healthy mental approach to test taking will also aid in other areas of life. Test anxiety affects more than just the actual test—it can be damaging to your mental health and even contribute to depression. It's important to beat test anxiety before it becomes a problem for more than testing.

> **Review Video: Test Anxiety and Depression**
> Visit mometrix.com/academy and enter code: 904704

Study Strategy

Being prepared for the test is necessary to combat anxiety, but what does being prepared look like? You may study for hours on end and still not feel prepared. What you need is a strategy for test prep. The next few pages outline our recommended steps to help you plan out and conquer the challenge of preparation.

Step 1: Scope Out the Test

Learn everything you can about the format (multiple choice, essay, etc.) and what will be on the test. Gather any study materials, course outlines, or sample exams that may be available. Not only will this help you to prepare, but knowing what to expect can help to alleviate test anxiety.

Step 2: Map Out the Material

Look through the textbook or study guide and make note of how many chapters or sections it has. Then divide these over the time you have. For example, if a book has 15 chapters and you have five days to study, you need to cover three chapters each day. Even better, if you have the time, leave an extra day at the end for overall review after you have gone through the material in depth.

If time is limited, you may need to prioritize the material. Look through it and make note of which sections you think you already have a good grasp on, and which need review. While you are studying, skim quickly through the familiar sections and take more time on the challenging parts. Write out your plan so you don't get lost as you go. Having a written plan also helps you feel more in control of the study, so anxiety is less likely to arise from feeling overwhelmed at the amount to cover. A sample plan may look like this:

- Day 1: Skim chapters 1–4, study chapter 5 (especially pages 31–33)
- Day 2: Study chapters 6–7, skim chapters 8–9
- Day 3: Skim chapter 10, study chapters 11–12 (especially pages 87–90)
- Day 4: Study chapters 13–15
- Day 5: Overall review (focus most on chapters 5, 6, and 12), take practice test

Step 3: Gather Your Tools

Decide what study method works best for you. Do you prefer to highlight in the book as you study and then go back over the highlighted portions? Or do you type out notes of the important information? Or is it helpful to make flashcards that you can carry with you? Assemble the pens, index cards, highlighters, post-it notes, and any other materials you may need so you won't be distracted by getting up to find things while you study.

If you're having a hard time retaining the information or organizing your notes, experiment with different methods. For example, try color-coding by subject with colored pens, highlighters, or post-it notes. If you learn better by hearing, try recording yourself reading your notes so you can listen while in the car, working out, or simply sitting at your desk. Ask a friend to quiz you from your flashcards, or try teaching someone the material to solidify it in your mind.

Step 4: Create Your Environment

It's important to avoid distractions while you study. This includes both the obvious distractions like visitors and the subtle distractions like an uncomfortable chair (or a too-comfortable couch that makes you want to fall asleep). Set up the best study environment possible: good lighting and a comfortable work area. If background music helps you focus, you may want to turn it on, but otherwise keep the room quiet. If you are using a computer to take notes, be sure you don't have any other windows open, especially applications like social media, games, or anything else that could distract you. Silence your phone and turn off notifications. Be sure to keep water close by so you stay hydrated while you study (but avoid unhealthy drinks and snacks).

Also, take into account the best time of day to study. Are you freshest first thing in the morning? Try to set aside some time then to work through the material. Is your mind clearer in the afternoon or evening? Schedule your study session then. Another method is to study at the same time of day that you will take the test, so that your brain gets used to working on the material at that time and will be ready to focus at test time.

Step 5: Study!

Once you have done all the study preparation, it's time to settle into the actual studying. Sit down, take a few moments to settle your mind so you can focus, and begin to follow your study plan. Don't give in to distractions or let yourself procrastinate. This is your time to prepare so you'll be ready to fearlessly approach the test. Make the most of the time and stay focused.

Of course, you don't want to burn out. If you study too long you may find that you're not retaining the information very well. Take regular study breaks. For example, taking five minutes out of every hour to walk briskly, breathing deeply and swinging your arms, can help your mind stay fresh.

As you get to the end of each chapter or section, it's a good idea to do a quick review. Remind yourself of what you learned and work on any difficult parts. When you feel that you've mastered the material, move on to the next part. At the end of your study session, briefly skim through your notes again.

But while review is helpful, cramming last minute is NOT. If at all possible, work ahead so that you won't need to fit all your study into the last day. Cramming overloads your brain with more information than it can process and retain, and your tired mind may struggle to recall even previously learned information when it is overwhelmed with last-minute study. Also, the urgent nature of cramming and the stress placed on your brain contribute to anxiety. You'll be more likely to go to the test feeling unprepared and having trouble thinking clearly.

So don't cram, and don't stay up late before the test, even just to review your notes at a leisurely pace. Your brain needs rest more than it needs to go over the information again. In fact, plan to finish your studies by noon or early afternoon the day before the test. Give your brain the rest of the day to relax or focus on other things, and get a good night's sleep. Then you will be fresh for the test and better able to recall what you've studied.

Step 6: Take a practice test

Many courses offer sample tests, either online or in the study materials. This is an excellent resource to check whether you have mastered the material, as well as to prepare for the test format and environment.

Check the test format ahead of time: the number of questions, the type (multiple choice, free response, etc.), and the time limit. Then create a plan for working through them. For example, if you have 30 minutes to take a 60-question test, your limit is 30 seconds per question. Spend less time on the questions you know well so that you can take more time on the difficult ones.

If you have time to take several practice tests, take the first one open book, with no time limit. Work through the questions at your own pace and make sure you fully understand them. Gradually work up to taking a test under test conditions: sit at a desk with all study materials put away and set a timer. Pace yourself to make sure you finish the test with time to spare and go back to check your answers if you have time.

After each test, check your answers. On the questions you missed, be sure you understand why you missed them. Did you misread the question (tests can use tricky wording)? Did you forget the information? Or was it something you hadn't learned? Go back and study any shaky areas that the practice tests reveal.

Taking these tests not only helps with your grade, but also aids in combating test anxiety. If you're already used to the test conditions, you're less likely to worry about it, and working through tests until you're scoring well gives you a confidence boost. Go through the practice tests until you feel comfortable, and then you can go into the test knowing that you're ready for it.

Test Tips

On test day, you should be confident, knowing that you've prepared well and are ready to answer the questions. But aside from preparation, there are several test day strategies you can employ to maximize your performance.

First, as stated before, get a good night's sleep the night before the test (and for several nights before that, if possible). Go into the test with a fresh, alert mind rather than staying up late to study.

Try not to change too much about your normal routine on the day of the test. It's important to eat a nutritious breakfast, but if you normally don't eat breakfast at all, consider eating just a protein bar. If you're a coffee drinker, go ahead and have your normal coffee. Just make sure you time it so that the caffeine doesn't wear off right in the middle of your test. Avoid sugary beverages, and drink enough water to stay hydrated but not so much that you need a restroom break 10 minutes into the test. If your test isn't first thing in the morning, consider going for a walk or doing a light workout before the test to get your blood flowing.

Allow yourself enough time to get ready, and leave for the test with plenty of time to spare so you won't have the anxiety of scrambling to arrive in time. Another reason to be early is to select a good seat. It's helpful to sit away from doors and windows, which can be distracting. Find a good seat, get out your supplies, and settle your mind before the test begins.

When the test begins, start by going over the instructions carefully, even if you already know what to expect. Make sure you avoid any careless mistakes by following the directions.

Then begin working through the questions, pacing yourself as you've practiced. If you're not sure on an answer, don't spend too much time on it, and don't let it shake your confidence. Either skip it and come back later, or eliminate as many wrong answers as possible and guess among the remaining ones. Don't dwell on these questions as you continue—put them out of your mind and focus on what lies ahead.

Be sure to read all of the answer choices, even if you're sure the first one is the right answer. Sometimes you'll find a better one if you keep reading. But don't second-guess yourself if you do immediately know the answer. Your gut instinct is usually right. Don't let test anxiety rob you of the information you know.

If you have time at the end of the test (and if the test format allows), go back and review your answers. Be cautious about changing any, since your first instinct tends to be correct, but make sure you didn't misread any of the questions or accidentally mark the wrong answer choice. Look over any you skipped and make an educated guess.

At the end, leave the test feeling confident. You've done your best, so don't waste time worrying about your performance or wishing you could change anything. Instead, celebrate the successful completion of this test. And finally, use this test to learn how to deal with anxiety even better next time.

> **Review Video: 5 Tips to Beat Test Anxiety**
> Visit mometrix.com/academy and enter code: 570656

Important Qualification

Not all anxiety is created equal. If your test anxiety is causing major issues in your life beyond the classroom or testing center, or if you are experiencing troubling physical symptoms related to your anxiety, it may be a sign of a serious physiological or psychological condition. If this sounds like your situation, we strongly encourage you to seek professional help.

Thank You

We at Mometrix would like to extend our heartfelt thanks to you, our friend and patron, for allowing us to play a part in your journey. It is a privilege to serve people from all walks of life who are unified in their commitment to building the best future they can for themselves.

The preparation you devote to these important testing milestones may be the most valuable educational opportunity you have for making a real difference in your life. We encourage you to put your heart into it—that feeling of succeeding, overcoming, and yes, conquering will be well worth the hours you've invested.

We want to hear your story, your struggles and your successes, and if you see any opportunities for us to improve our materials so we can help others even more effectively in the future, please share that with us as well. **The team at Mometrix would be absolutely thrilled to hear from you!** So please, send us an email (support@mometrix.com) and let's stay in touch.

If you'd like some additional help, check out these other resources we offer for your exam:

http://MometrixFlashcards.com/InpatientObstetric

Additional Bonus Material

Due to our efforts to try to keep this book to a manageable length, we've created a link that will give you access to all of your additional bonus material.

Please visit **https://www.mometrix.com/bonus948/inpobstnurse** to access the information.